Contents

The psychological care of medical patients

A practical guide

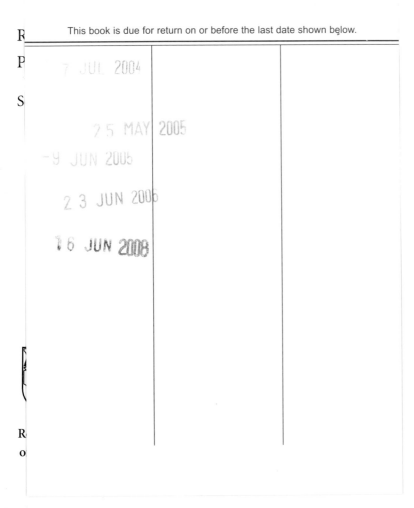

Royal College of Physicians of London
11 St Andrews Place, London NW1 4LE
Registered Charity No 210508

Royal College of Psychiatrists
17 Belgrave Square, London SW1X 8PG
Registered Charity No 228636

Royal College of Psychiatrists Council Report No: CR108
Royal College of Psychiatrists review date: October 2007

ISBN 1 86016 178 2

Text editing and layout by the Publications Department
of the Royal College of Physicians
Cover design: Merriton Sharp
Typeset by Dan-Set Graphics, Telford, Shropshire
Printed in Great Britain by Sarum ColourView Group, Salisbury, Wiltshire

Working party members

Dr G Lloyd (*Chairman*) MD FRCP FRCPsych
   Consultant Liaison Psychiatrist, Royal Free Hospital, London

Mr A Cairns LIB
   Divisional Director, Leeds Teaching Hospitals Trust

Dr KM Checinski MB BS MRCPsych
   Senior Lecturer in Addictive Behaviour, St George's Hospital Medical School;
   Hononary Consultant, Surrey Oaklands NHS Trust

Dr M Donaghy DPhil FRCP
   Reader in Clinical Neurology, University of Oxford;
   Honorary Consultant in Neurology, Radcliffe Infirmary, Oxford

Dr EJ Feldman MA DM(Oxon) MRCPsych
   Consultant Liaison Psychiatrist, John Radcliffe Hospital, Oxford;
   Honorary Senior Clinical Lecturer, University of Oxford

Dr DR Forsyth MA FRCP
   Consultant Geriatrician, Addenbrooke's NHS Trust Hospital, Cambridge;
   Chairman, British Geriatrics Society Special Interest Group on Cerebral
   Ageing and Mental Health

Dr JSR Gibbs MD FRCP
   Senior Lecturer in Cardiology, National Heart and Lung Institute, Faculty of
   Medicine, Imperial College of Science, Technology and Medicine;
   Honorary Consultant, Hammersmith Hospital, London

Mrs C Gratus BA MBA
   Vice-Chair, Clinical Oncology Patient Liaison Group, Royal College of
   Radiologists

Professor E Guthrie MB ChB MRCPsych MSc MD
   Professor of Psychological Medicine and Medical Psychotherapy,
   School of Psychiatry and Behavioural Science, University of Manchester

Mr A Harrison RMN DipN MSc
   Consultant Nurse (Liaison Psychiatry), Avon & Wiltshire Mental Health
   Partnership NHS Trust, Bath; Visiting Fellow, University of the West of
   England, Bristol

Professor K Hawton DSc FRCPsych
   Consultant Psychiatrist, Director of Centre for Suicide Research,
   University of Oxford, Warneford Hospital, Oxford

Dr AC Higgitt BSc MB BS MD FRCPsych

Consultant Psychiatrist, Senior Policy Adviser, Mental Health Services Branch, Department of Health

Dr JD Holmes MA MD MRCP MRCPsych

Senior Lecturer in Liaison Psychiatry of Old Age, University of Leeds

Mr S Lennox BSc RGN RMN

Head of Clinical Development, Epsom and St Helier NHS Trust

Professor MB McIllmurray DM FRCP

Macmillan Consultant in Medical Oncology, Morecambe Bay Hospitals NHS Trust

Dr S Michie MPhil DPhil FBPsS

Reader in Clinical Health Psychology, Centre for Outcomes Research and Effectiveness, Department of Psychology, University College London

Professor RE Pounder MD DSc(Med) FRCP

Clinical Vice-President, Royal College of Physicians

Professor L Turner-Stokes DM FRCP

Herbert Dunhill Chair of Rehabilitation, King's College London; Consultant Physician in Rehabilitation Medicine, Director, Regional Rehabilitation Unit, Northwick Park Hospital

Professor J Weinman BA PhD CPsychol FBPsS DSc(Hon)

Professor in Psychology as applied to Medicine, Unit of Psychology, GKT School of Medicine, King's College London

Foreword

The importance of the psychological dimension of medical practice is now firmly established. Hospital doctors, like their colleagues in primary care, recognise that in many patients medical illness is accompanied by psychological distress that also requires intervention. Other patients referred with somatic symptoms are found to have little or no physical pathology but are manifesting psychological distress in physical ways. General hospital doctors also treat a large number of patients following deliberate self-harm or with complications of drug and alcohol misuse. For such patients, the general hospital is often a way into psychiatric care.

Physicians therefore need to be able to identify patients with significant psychological problems, and to distinguish between those who need to be referred for specialist psychiatric or psychological assessment, and those they can treat themselves. For the latter group, physicians obviously also need to know how to provide appropriate psychological support. This report aims to provide practical guidance on these matters for physicians and other clinical staff who work in general hospitals. It updates and complements an earlier report, *The psychological care of medical patients: recognition of need and service provision*, published in 1995.

Sensitive communication skills are crucial if patients' psychological problems are to be identified and managed successfully. Liaison psychiatry services are gradually being developed in general hospitals but are often rudimentary and largely confined to the treatment of patients who deliberately self-harm. At a time when general psychiatry is concentrating on the treatment of chronically ill patients in the community, it is important to ensure that healthcare commissioners are aware of the need for a multidisciplinary liaison psychiatry team in each general hospital. This report argues persuasively for this development.

January 2003

Professor Carol Black,
President, Royal College of Physicians of London

Dr Mike Shooter,
President, Royal College of Psychiatrists

Executive summary and recommendations

Doctors are increasingly aware of the importance of developing good communication skills and of attending to their patients' psychological symptoms. This second joint report of the Royal College of Physicians and Royal College of Psychiatrists aims to highlight the importance of addressing the psychological dimension of medical practice and to foster the development of services designed to improve the psychological care of medical patients. The latter target is best achieved by establishing a multidisciplinary liaison psychiatry service in every general hospital.

Although most people adjust well to the limitations imposed by their illness, a significant proportion find that their coping mechanisms are overwhelmed. The high prevalence of psychiatric disorders in general hospital patients is now well established. Depression, anxiety disorders, delirium and substance misuse are particularly common, and deliberate self-harm accounts for approximately 140,000 presentations to hospitals in England and Wales each year. Physicians need to be able to identify these problems, to arrange basic psychological care and to know when to refer patients to specialist psychiatric and psychological services. Depression and other psychiatric disorders have often been regarded as inevitable and understandable responses to illness and therefore not amenable to treatment. This opinion is no longer sustainable. Patients with significant and persistent psychological symptoms respond well to psychological or pharmacological treatments. Therapeutic interventions are also effective for managing patients with problems of alcohol misuse, those who present after episodes of self-harm and those who somatise their problems.

Recommendations

The Working Party makes the following recommendations to promote the psychological care of medical patients in general hospitals:

1. Liaison psychiatry services should be established in all general hospitals that are commissioned to provide comprehensive medical care for a defined population. The service should be multidisciplinary and include nurses, clinical psychologists, social workers and trainee psychiatrists, led by a consultant psychiatrist with special training in liaison psychiatry. Clinicians in other specialties should have ready access to the expertise of a liaison psychiatry team.

2 Teaching hospitals require increased staffing levels to cope with demands
   from tertiary medical services. Some hospitals have developed special
   liaison services to manage patients following deliberate self-harm and those
   with alcohol and drug problems. These developments should be supported.

3 Communication skills are fundamental to good clinical care and facilitate
   detection of psychological problems. These skills should be taught during
   postgraduate medical training and actively maintained throughout a
   professional career. Physicians could also gain valuable and relevant
   experience by spending six months at senior house officer level in
   psychiatry.

4 Training should be provided to enable physicians to apply basic
   psychological treatments, to recognise the indications for prescribing
   psychotropic drugs, and to manage patients suffering from alcohol and
   drug misuse.

5 Simple protocols should be developed for the detection and management
   of common psychological problems by general hospital staff.

6 Referral of patients to a liaison psychiatry service should be uncomplicated,
   with clear guidelines as to who should be referred.

7 There should be good channels of communication within the general
   hospital and with community services with regard to psychiatric as well as
   physical health.

8 Liaison psychiatry departments require adequate space for clinical work
   together with space for secretarial staff and support facilities to provide
   computerised record-keeping, thus enabling audit and clinical research to
   be undertaken.

9 Clinicians should be familiar with the principles of common law and the
   Mental Health Act 1983 as they apply to general hospital practice. Hospital
   trusts should arrange appropriate training for doctors and non-medical
   staff, including security staff.

10 The separation of mental health services and acute hospital trusts creates
   difficulties for liaison psychiatry, and management arrangements will vary
   according to established local practice. To ensure optimum delivery, a
   liaison psychiatry service should be managed within an acute hospital trust,
   alongside other medical specialties.

11 Funding for liaison psychiatry should be provided by those specialties that
   use the service. Recognition of this funding should be incorporated into all
   service agreements between acute hospital trusts and their commissioners.

1 | Introduction

SUMMARY

▶ The report addresses the particular psychological problems experienced by patients attending general hospitals. It aims to encourage clinicians to develop skills of good psychological care and to promote a psychological component in organisational development.

▶ This is a practical guide which outlines the common psychiatric syndromes and advises on their recognition and management.

▶ Communications skills are fundamentally important and are given special consideration in the report.

▶ Emphasis is also placed on the need for doctors to be familiar with the Mental Health Act 1983 and common law as they apply to general hospital practice.

▶ The case for developing liaison psychiatry services in all general hospitals has gained ground following the shift of mental health care towards a community-based service.

The psychological welfare of medical patients is attracting increasing attention. Becoming physically ill is a stressful experience. Whilst most people adjust well to the limitations imposed by their condition, a significant number develop some form of psychological disorder secondary to their physical disease. Other patients present with physical symptoms for which no adequate medical explanation can be established and in many the symptoms are found to be the result of a hitherto unrecognised psychological problem. Several government reports in England and Wales have emphasised the need for medical patients to have access to psychiatric and psychological services.[1,2] The first joint report from the Royal Colleges of Physicians and Psychiatrists highlighted the nature of the problems and made recommendations for the provision of psychological care in general hospitals.[3] The present report updates the earlier report in the light of recent developments in treatment, health service organisation and medical law.

1.1   Aims of the report

The aims of this report are similar to those of its predecessor in addressing the particular psychological problems likely to be experienced by patients attending general hospitals, either in secondary or tertiary services. It is specifically concerned with adult patients under the care of physicians in any of the recognised medical specialties, but its principles are relevant to other branches of medicine. It is also relevant to adults with learning difficulties although it does not address their needs specifically, for which the reader is referred to a separate report in England[4] and similar reports in Scotland[5] and Wales.[6] This report does not cover the needs of children and adolescents.

We wish to encourage all hospital staff to develop skills of good psychological care and to be able to assess and manage their patients' psychological problems. We also wish to promote a psychological component in organisational development which includes staff education and support, and hospital design. The report will therefore be relevant not only to physicians but also to clinical psychologists, nurses, managers and other professionals who work with medical patients in general hospitals.

This is essentially a practical guide for clinicians. It outlines the common psychiatric syndromes encountered in day-to-day practice and advises on how these can be recognised. Special consideration is given to developing communication skills, which are crucially important in the provision of better treatment and general care, and in the detection of psychiatric disorders. Also, patients now expect more open communication with their doctors. They want more information about their health problems and expect to be involved in decisions concerning their treatment. For many patients the role of a carer is also important. Doctors need to be aware of these expectations and to be able to provide support and information according to patients' needs, which often change with time. We have also given special attention to the use of the Mental Health Act 1983 and common law in the general hospital. Recent case law has clarified the doctor's responsibility in assessing mental capacity and providing treatment for those who are unable to give informed consent. In future, liaison psychiatrists are likely to become involved more often in advising their colleagues when a patient's competence to refuse or consent to treatment is in doubt, or when a patient wishes to die by terminating life-support treatment.

Physicians successfully treat considerable psychiatric morbidity in their patients and do so without the assistance of psychiatrists or any other mental health professionals. It is highly appropriate that this should continue. The various treatment options available to the clinician are reviewed here with reference to recent publications establishing the effectiveness of psychological and pharmacological treatments. It is clear that therapeutic nihilism is misplaced: treatments work.

By highlighting the prevalence of psychiatric disorder in general hospitals and the real benefits to patients if this is managed appropriately, we hope to see a sustained development of liaison services throughout the country. The report sets out the clearest possible case for ensuring that the psychological care of medical patients is given a much higher priority within the service agreements between acute hospital trusts and their commissioners.

1.2　Psychological and psychiatric problems in the general hospital

The more common psychological and psychiatric problems seen in general hospital practice are:

▶ physical and psychiatric comorbidity

▶ medically unexplained symptoms

▶ deliberate self-harm

▶ drug and alcohol misuse

▶ acute organic disorders

▶ behavioural problems (eg non-adherence to treatment, lack of capacity to consent).

Patients with these problems often have complex needs, requiring the co-ordinated help of a multidisciplinary medical team. Only a minority require referral to a mental health professional. The report provides guidance as to when referral to a psychiatrist or psychologist is appropriate, although this cannot be specified precisely because much depends on local facilities and the clinician's own interest and expertise. When specialist mental health management is required, it is best if this is delivered by a liaison psychiatry service which should include liaison nurses, clinical psychologists and social workers in addition to consultant and trainee psychiatrists. The original report made specific recom-mendations about the staffing of a liaison service and that advice has been followed in many hospitals. There has been a steady expansion of posts in liaison psychiatry, health psychology and liaison nursing, although developments have not been uniform throughout the country: some hospitals, particularly district general hospitals, continue to have rudimentary liaison services often amounting to no more than an assessment service for patients following episodes of deliber-ate self-harm. In view of the accumulating evidence for therapeutic effectiveness, this is an area of healthcare delivery where failure to provide an available and responsive service can no longer be justified.

1.3   Identifying patients and referral for treatment

Much has been written about the identification of patients who have developed a
psychiatric disorder but who have been referred to a physician because of
concurrent somatic symptoms, whether or not these symptoms are the manifestations of organic pathology. It is generally acknowledged that psychiatric disorders
are much more difficult to detect when masked by somatic complaints and
therefore such patients' psychological problems are less likely to be recognised and
treated. A theoretical remedy to this problem is to use one or more screening
instruments in the shape of questionnaires devised to detect depression, anxiety or
other psychological symptoms. High scores will identify patients with psychiatric
disorders for whom appropriate treatment can then be arranged. Unfortunately
such an approach has not been vindicated by controlled trials,[7,8] and the routine
use of screening instruments cannot be recommended in general hospital practice.
Identification of those with psychiatric disorders continues to be based on clinical
assessment involving a carefully taken history and an evaluation of the patient's
mental state, supplemented by other sources of information provided by the
general practitioner, relatives and friends. The physician thus has a pivotal role in
the diagnosis of psychiatric disorder.

It is important that the training of physicians and other clinical staff emphasises
the development of communication and interviewing skills. Postgraduate medical
education is encouraging doctors to specialise at an early stage in their careers
and training schemes lack the flexibility to enable experience of other specialties
to be acquired. We believe that many physicians would gain valuable and
relevant experience if they were able to spend six months at senior house officer
level in psychiatry. Conversely, trainee psychiatrists would benefit by spending an
equivalent period in a medical post. The recent introduction of psychiatry posts at
pre-registration house officer level is a welcome development which enables more
doctors to obtain experience of psychiatry after qualifying.

Since the establishment of separate mental health trusts, the case for the
development of liaison psychiatry services has gained ground.[9] Psychiatry and
psychology have moved their focus of operation from hospitals into the community
and many general psychiatrists currently spend most of their time in community
mental health centres or treating patients in their homes. They have little time for
general hospital work, and nor do they have the required expertise. Acute trusts and
mental health trusts will need to develop clear responses to this new organisational
context. It will be essential to ensure that liaison psychiatry services are placed at
the forefront of the relationship between acute and mental health trusts if medical
patients are not to fall into an organisational vacuum.

References

1   Department of Health. *National Service Framework for older people.* London: DH, 2001.

2   Department of Health. *The NHS cancer plan: a plan for investment, a plan for reform.* Leeds: DH, 2000.

3   Royal College of Physicians and Royal College of Psychiatrists. *Psychological care of medical of medical patients: recognition and service provision.* A joint working party report. London: RCP, 1995.

4   Department of Health. *Valuing people: a new strategy for learning disability for the 21st century.* London: DH, 2001.

5   Scottish Executive Health Department. *The same as you.* Edinburgh: SEHD, 2001.

6   National Assembly of Wales. *Fulfilling the promises.* Cardiff: NAW, 2001.

7   Levenson JL, Hamer RM, Rossiter LF. A randomised controlled trial of psychiatric consultation guided by screening in general medical inpatients. *Am J Psychiatry* 1992;**149**:631–7.

8   Gater RA, Goldberg DP, Evanson JM, Lawson K *et al.* Detection and treatment of psychiatric illness in a general medical ward: a modified cost-benefit analysis. *J Psychosom Res* 1998;**45**:437–8.

9   Lloyd GG, Mayou RA. Liaison psychiatry or psychological medicine? *Br J Psychiatry* (in press).

Further reading

Guthrie E, Creed F (eds). *Seminars in liaison psychiatry.* London: Gaskell, 1996.

Peveler R, Feldman E, Friedman T (eds). *Liaison psychiatry: planning services for specialist settings.* London: Gaskell, 2001.

2 | Communication and psychological assessment

SUMMARY

▶ Good communication is associated with patient satisfaction, adherence to health advice, improved health outcome and fewer complaints.

▶ Doctors should elicit patients' beliefs and concerns, listen to patients, and encourage active involvement in decision-making and in managing their health.

▶ Clear, simple written and verbal information should be given early, often and appropriately. Patients' comprehension and recall should be checked and they should be encouraged to ask questions.

▶ Patient distress should be acknowledged and responded to appropriately, allowing time to understand reasons for anxiety, depression or anger.

▶ Patients' individual characteristics and the social and cultural context should be recognised and understood.

Effective communication is necessary to ensure that patients' problems and concerns are understood by those providing care, and that relevant information, advice and treatment are understood, recalled and acted upon by patients. Doctors are often reluctant to give patients information. Up to 50% of patients are critical of the communication aspects of their hospital care, even when clinicians think they have made special efforts to communicate well.[1] Patients complain that clinicians do not appear to be interested in their presenting problems or in their concerns about them. This may risk delaying diagnosis and reduce patients' confidence in the healthcare system. A third area of dissatisfaction is that patients feel that they are not sufficiently involved in decision-making about their healthcare.

Clinicians find it more difficult to communicate with some groups of patients, for example those with mental health or drug problems. Also, clinicians attending communication training courses found that the most difficult patients to manage were those from ethnic minorities, the young, adolescents, elderly people, those with young children and those with whom they personally identified.[2] The most common problems they experienced were imparting complex information, eliciting and dealing with psychosocial concerns, reacting appropriately to patients' emotions, dealing with angry relatives, breaking bad news and obtaining informed consent.

2.1   The benefits of good communication

Good communication enhances clinical outcome in the following areas:

▸ cognitive (knowledge, understanding and recall)

▸ affective (satisfaction/distress)

▸ behavioural (adherence to advice).

Studies have shown that, on average, no more than half of the information given to patients is recalled. Satisfaction is a broad indicator of the patient's affective response to a consultation. It is also associated with cooperation and adherence to advice, improved health status and fewer malpractice claims. The clinician has a key role in both understanding the patient perspective and empowering patients to take an active part in managing their own care.[3]

Poor communication is a common reason for non-adherence to advice. Patients may not have understood or recalled the information given or they may have beliefs which conflict with the advice but which were never elicited by the clinician.

The main benefits of good communication with patients are summarised in Box 2.1.

Box 2.1   Benefits of good communication

▸ Patient knowledge, understanding and recall are improved
▸ Anxiety is reduced and satisfaction with care increased
▸ Adherence to health advice is increased
▸ There are fewer malpractice claims

2.2   Providing information

In general, patients want more information than they are given. Since patients vary in their existing knowledge, the amount and type of information they want and their expectations of the consultation, it is important to discuss these with them. It is also essential to check the comprehension and recall of relevant information with patients at regular intervals. A common communication problem is the use of jargon and technical terms. Verbal information should be backed up with written information, and both should be easy to understand. Written information should include copies of correspondence that summarise what has been covered in the consultation. Routine copying of correspondence is considered to be good professional practice. Tape-recordings of consultations and website addresses are other helpful forms of information, although website information varies considerably in its accuracy and usefulness. Providing patients with a copy of their records can be another useful way of communicating, as can encouraging patients to write down questions for clinicians.

Understanding and recall are impaired if patients are anxious, if information is detailed or complex, and if a large amount of information is given at one time.[4] It is therefore important to give the most important information (for example, advice that should be followed) at the beginning of the consultation and again at the end. If information is made specific, presented in categories and emphasised, it is more likely to be recalled and acted on.

The physical context of giving information should be such that patients feel comfortable, both psychologically and physically. They need to feel that their privacy and confidentiality are respected. The consultation should be free from distractions and interruptions. Ward settings rarely achieve this. When interviewing patients, issues of confidentiality should be discussed, including any limits of confidentiality.

Box 2.2   Essentials of good communication

Good communication requires:
▶ expressing interest in the patient
▶ eliciting patients' beliefs and concerns
▶ acknowledging and responding to patients' distress
▶ avoiding jargon and overly complex information
▶ a collaborative and empowering approach
▶ privacy and confidentiality

Increasingly, health information is given not as definite diagnoses, but as risk estimates. Screening tests, by their nature, only give probabilistic information. Patients are expected to understand a bewildering variety of risk figures, given numerically in different ways or in verbal phrases, given in absolute or relative terms, and given in positive or negative frames (eg 'the glass is half full or half empty'). Patients are expected to weigh up different kinds of risks in making their choices. For example, women receiving a positive prenatal screening result are faced with understanding the meaning of the positive result as well as the risks associated with continuing or terminating the pregnancy. Those receiving a negative result are faced with understanding the meaning of a residual risk. Counselling before and after such screening tests should therefore be provided routinely.

Patients feel more satisfied if clinicians accompany information-giving with social conversation, show positive verbal and non-verbal behaviour and build up a partnership with them.[5] This is one aspect of a style of communication that will benefit patients (see Box 2.2). Clinicians should also be aware of their own attitudes and behaviour towards patients. Those who see patients as having caused or exacerbated their condition through their own behaviour or neglect may be less committed, motivated and sympathetic towards them.

Good communication within teams and between clinicians is also essential if patients are to receive a consistent message from the many people they are likely to meet in the healthcare system. If information is inconsistent or contradictory, this will cause distress, undermine adherence, result in lack of confidence in the team and increase the likelihood of complaints.

2.3   Language difficulties and disabilities

In addition to these general principles, some groups of patients have specific needs. Linguistic understanding should not be assumed, but established; a reluctance to speak may reflect limitations of expression in the English language. Patients not fluent in English should be provided with translated written material and an interpreter should be present during the consultation. Clinicians should be aware of any deficits the patient might have and adjust their communication accordingly. Cognitive deficits are often not detected (see Box 2.3).

2.4   Listening to patients

Good communication is a two-way process: it requires both effective talking and effective listening (see Box 2.4). Patients have their own beliefs about their bodies, health and illnesses. Successful communication requires that clinicians elicit these and try to correct misconceptions. Information and advice should be given within patients' own framework and understanding. This patient-centred approach allows for agreement over the nature of the problem and the best course of action. Patients then feel more satisfied and are more likely to follow advice. Despite this, patient-centred communication is seldom used in clinical practice, and only a minority of patient concerns are elicited.[6]

A key issue in effective communication concerns patients' cultural background. Different cultures have different beliefs about health, illness, health services and

Box 2.3 Specific advice for different disabilities

Visual impairment

▶ Adjust positioning/lighting so that light is on your face

▶ Avoid bright lights/window behind you which will put you in silhouette

▶ Use a large font for written information

Hearing loss

▶ Remove background noise – turn off radios etc

▶ Speak clearly and avoid long sentences

▶ Do not shout

▶ Face the patient when you talk to him/her and do not cover your mouth with your hand

▶ Write things down

▶ Use amplifiers and, where appropriate, use sign language or interpreters

Dysphasia/dysarthria

▶ Establish the patient's level of comprehension and of expression

▶ Use short sentences

▶ Use single words where possible

▶ Encourage yes/no responses only

▶ Communicate with pictures or other aids

▶ Consider using gestures

▶ Find out whether written cues help

▶ Enlist the help of a speech and language therapist if in doubt

▶ Don't pretend to understand your patient if you don't

Cognitive deficits

▶ Ensure that you have engaged the patient's attention

▶ Use the patient's name to refocus his/her attention if necessary

▶ Use simple language and short sentences

▶ Ask patients to feed back to you what they have understood as you go along

▶ Enlist the help of a nurse/key-worker who can reiterate the information for them, using the same terminology

▶ Write information down

treatments. These often stem from religious beliefs. If clinicians are to engage patients from a variety of ethnic groups, to understand them and be listened to by them, they need to have knowledge of relevant cultural and religious beliefs and practices. Different social groups may also have their own 'slang' or 'street

> **Box 2.4   Steps to achieve patient-centred communication**
>
> ▶ Elicit patients' beliefs and concerns about illness and treatment
> ▶ Facilitate patients' active involvement in consultation by asking open-ended questions, seeking their views, and allowing time for and discussion of patients' questions
> ▶ Encourage active participation in discussion and management of their own health
> ▶ Ensure that patients participate in goal-setting and in agreeing methods for achieving goals
> ▶ Help patients determine methods for monitoring and, if necessary, modifying goals and related behaviours

language'. It is important that clinicians ask for clarification if they are not sure whether they have correctly understood the meaning of unfamiliar words or phrases.

The non-verbal behaviour ('body language' and facial expression) of patients may provide important information about their mood and concerns. Similarly, the non-verbal behaviour of clinicians conveys messages about their level of interest in the problem and attitudes to the patient. If patients perceive the clinician as unsympathetic, they are less likely to listen to what is said to them, to provide information about their concerns or to follow advice given.

Many patients are reluctant to ask for information or to complain. This partly reflects a general expectation that 'good' patients are those who do what they are told and make minimal demands on others. They may also be afraid of showing their ignorance. The clinician needs to keep these factors in mind in making patients feel at ease, enabling them to say what is on their mind, to ask questions and to complain if they are dissatisfied.

2.5   Involving patients in decision-making

Patients differ in the extent to which they wish to be involved in treatment decisions. However, the majority prefer a collaborative approach, and offering choice of treatment and following patients' preferences have been found to reduce anxiety and depression. Thus, informed choice and consent are not just abstract principles, but are associated with good psychological outcomes, both emotional and behavioural. Informed choice refers to a decision that is based on relevant knowledge and is consistent with the decision-maker's values (see Box 2.5).[7]

Box 2.5   Steps to achieving informed choice/consent

▶ Establish current knowledge and understanding

▶ Fill in gaps in knowledge and provide written information

▶ Ask about relevant attitudes and values

▶ Present options and ask about initial preferences

▶ Facilitate discussion of options in the context of relevant information, and patients' attitudes and values

▶ If possible, allow patients time to reflect on the options and to discuss them with others

▶ Engage in shared decision-making to reach an agreed and acceptable decision

▶ Ensure that written consent is gained only after all the above steps have been taken

2.6   Managing uncertainty and breaking bad news

Common mistakes when giving bad news are to give patients insufficient information about their prognosis and to avoid exploring their concerns, worries and associated feelings.[8] This means that patients remain preoccupied with their worries, which have not been addressed, and selectively recall negative phrases, even when positive statements were also made by the clinician. One of the strongest predictors of later anxiety and depression is the number and severity of patients' unresolved concerns.[9]

When there is no clear diagnosis or prognosis physicians are required to give uncertain information that is based on probability. Particular skills are needed to convey such information in a way that patients can understand and use in making decisions and future plans (see Box 2.6).

Patients' responses to bad news are highly variable and unpredictable. They may express their distress as extreme anger, which may include anger towards the 'messenger'. If this occurs, the clinician–patient relationship is vulnerable and must be preserved by patience and understanding. Clinicians should be prepared for such reactions and be confident in their skills to manage them. Often it is valuable to discuss a diagnosis with the patient in stages, preferably in the presence of a close relative.

The main reasons that clinicians avoid dealing with the emotional aspects of bad news are:

▶ lack of training

▶ fear of increasing patients' distress

> **Box 2.6   Communicating risk and uncertain information**
>
> ▸ Ascertain current understanding and knowledge
> ▸ Introduce concept of medicine as an inexact science, with many clinical situations having a degree of uncertainty attached to them
> ▸ Use different forms of presentation, eg numbers, pictures, analogies
> ▸ Be aware of the power of framing information (eg whether the glass is half full or half empty)
> ▸ Check patients' understanding of the information given
> ▸ Provide opportunity for future questions and discussion, particularly if there are likely to be changes in the clinical situation or patient perspective

> ▸ lack of emotional and practical support from colleagues
> ▸ concern for one's own emotional survival.

Two of the key principles of giving bad news well are to tailor the information to what the patient wishes and is ready to hear, and to give enough time to the process (see Box 2.7). This will allow the patient to take in the information, without provoking denial or overwhelming distress. A third principle is to avoid withholding information because a relative insists that the patient is unable to handle the news. Such collusion has adverse psychological consequences, both for the patient and relatives. On the other hand, a patient's expressed view about what they do not want to hear should be respected. A fourth principle is to acknowledge distress, to explore reasons for it and to check that the patient would like to continue the discussion.[10]

> **Box 2.7   Breaking bad news (adapted from Ref 10)**
>
> ▸ Find out what the patient knows and wants to know
> ▸ Allow enough time and give information in stages
> ▸ Give full information to patients and important others
> ▸ Understand and help patients manage their distress

2.7   Stressful medical procedures

The stress of medical procedures can be reduced by providing information to reduce patients' uncertainty. This includes information about the various procedures that will take place at different stages and information about what is likely to be felt. Pain and discomfort are less distressing if they are expected. It is also helpful to give patients advice about behaviours and cognitive coping procedures that will reduce unpleasant sensations and increase relaxation.

2.8   Developing communication skills

A key skill is that of 'active' listening which includes developing rapport, using open-ended questions early in the consultation, appropriate eye contact and other facilitatory responses to help the patient talk (see Box 2.8). Another basic skill is that of summarising and developing a shared understanding of the presenting problem. Dealing with distressed patients and giving bad news require clinicians to deal with their own emotions in these situations. Training in all these skills is best done interactively, using role play, video feedback and time to address difficult issues.

Identifying patients who are psychologically distressed requires:

- making good eye contact at the outset
- clarifying patients' complaints
- responding to verbal cues suggestive of emotional distress
- asking questions about patients' feelings
- enquiring about the situation at home
- making supportive comments
- handling interruptions well
- maintaining eye contact.

A randomised controlled trial of general practitioners being trained in 'problem defining' or 'emotion handling' behaviours found that only half of those receiving training were able to recognise patients with high emotional distress.[11]

There have also been a number of interventions used with patients before their consultations. Most have aimed to increase their level of participation in the consultation to ensure that their own concerns are dealt with and that information

---

Box 2.8   Active listening skills

- Develop rapport
- Facilitate dialogue, eg by using open-ended questions and keeping good eye-contact
- Summarise and agree a shared view of the problem and how to deal with it
- Show ability to detect and respond appropriately to patient distress

provided by the clinician is clearly understood. These has been shown to be effective and to be associated with improved health outcome.[12]

2.9   Stress and communication

Just as patients are less effective communicators when anxious, so clinicians are less effective communicators when stressed. Unfortunately, high levels of stress are commonly experienced by clinicians, much of it caused by heavy workloads, time pressures and responsibility for people's lives.[13] One of the most stressful situations can be facing angry patients and relatives, but the behaviour of clinicians can help to defuse anger and conflict (see Box 2.9).

Box 2.9   Handling anger and conflict

▸ Express your point of view in a non-threatening way (verbally and non-verbally)
▸ Listen to other people, and summarise what they have said to show that they have been heard
▸ Be specific – keep the issues as circumscribed as possible
▸ Use a 'grain of truth' approach – find something positive to acknowledge in what the other is saying
▸ Emphasise areas of agreement, eg shared goals
▸ Negotiate for compromise – don't back the other into a corner
▸ Build a future review into the situation

Stress impairs communication, which causes more stress, creating a vicious circle. Reducing stress requires a twin-track approach, working at both individual and organisational levels.[14] At an individual level, health workers can undergo training or seek support to help them identify the causes of their stress and increase their buffers against the adverse effects of stress. At an organisational level, employers can identify situations that put their staff at risk of experiencing high levels of stress and work to change these. They can also make structural changes that give more support and control to staff, both of which have been found to reduce stress associated with high workloads.

2.10   Brief psychiatric or psychological assessment

It is possible for clinicians to make a brief psychiatric or psychological assessment in 5–10 minutes (see Table 2.1). The main purpose of this should be to establish the presence of a psychological problem or psychiatric disorder and to determine any major current risk. It is also helpful to check whether other important factors (eg alcohol abuse) have been identified.

Table 2.1 Elements of a brief psychological/psychiatric assessment

Beliefs and adjustment to illness	Major fears or worries (do they seem out of proportion?) Evidence of adjustment
Current symptoms, eg depression, anxiety	Duration and severity Relationship to physical illness (ie preceded or followed onset of physical condition)
Cognitive function	Orientation, level of consciousness, concentration and memory
Risk	Any active thoughts of self-harm Threatening or abusive behaviour
Biological symptoms	Likely relationship to physical illness (ie are symptoms such as insomnia, anorexia and weight loss attributable to the illness?)
Level of functioning	In relation to physical disability (better, normal or poorer than expected)
Known current stressors or important past events	For example redundancy, a recent bereavement, or a history of sexual abuse
Previous history	Previous contact with psychiatric or pyschological services
Alcohol intake Drugs	Evidence of harmful or hazardous drinking Evidence of illicit drug-taking
Current medication	Any prescribed drugs which cause depression, anxiety, confusion or psychosis

2.11 Regular observation

If a psychiatric disorder is suspected in a patient already in hospital, the nursing staff should be asked to devise a care plan to include routine observation of the following: fluid intake, diet, weight, sleep, social interaction with visitors and other patients, mood, and any unusual or inappropriate behaviour.

If suicidal ideas have been elicited, patients should be asked not to leave the ward and should be observed regularly. An urgent psychiatric opinion should be requested.

References

1   Weinman J. Health care. In Johnston DW and Johnston M (eds), *Health psychology*, vol 8, *Introduction to comprehensive clinical psychology*. Oxford: Elsevier Science, 2001.

2   Fallowfield L, Lipkin M, Hall A. Teaching senior oncologists communication skills: results from phase one of a comprehensive program in the UK. *J Clin Oncol* 1998;**16**:1961–8.

3   Michie S, Mannion J, Weinman J (in press). Patient-centredness in chronic illness: what is it and does it matter? *Patient Educ Couns* (in press).

4   Ley P. *Communication with patients*. London: Croom-Helm, 1988.

5   Roter D, Hall JA. Studies of doctor patient interaction. *Ann Rev Public Health* 1989;**10**:163–80.

6   Maguire P. Improving communication with cancer patients. *Eur J Cancer* 1999;**35**:1415–22.

7   O'Connor A, O'Brien Pallas LL. Decisional conflict. In McFarlane GK, McFarlane EA (eds), *Nursing diagnosis and intervention*. Toronto: Mosby, 1998:486–96.

8   Maguire, P. Barriers to psychological care of the dying. *BMJ* 1985:**291**:1711–13.

9   Parle M, Jones B, Maguire P. Maladaptive coping and affective disorders in cancer patients. *Psychol Med* 1996;**26**:736–44.

10 Maguire, P. Breaking bad news. In Baum A., Newman S, Weinman J, West R, McManus C (eds), *Cambridge handbook of psychology, health and medicine*. Cambridge: Cambridge University Press, 1997:273–5.

11 Goldberg DP, Steele JJ, Smith C, Spivey L. Training family doctors to recognize psychiatric illness with increased accuracy. *Lancet* 1980; **ii**:521–3.

12 Greenfield S, Kaplan S, Ware JE. Expanding patient involvement in care: effects on patient outcomes. *Ann Intern Med* 1985;**102**:520–28.

13 Williams S, Michie S, Pattani S. *Improving the health of the NHS workforce.* A Nuffield Trust Report of the Partnership on the Health of the NHS Workforce. London: Nuffield Trust, 1998.

14 Michie S (2002). Causes and management of stress at work. *Occup Environ Med* **59**:67–72.

Further reading

Bayne R, Nicolson P, Horton I (eds). *Counselling and communication skills for medical and health practitioners*. Leicester: BPS Books,1998.

Lloyd M, Bor R. *Communication skills for medicine*. Edinburgh: Churchill Livingstone, 1996.

Royal College of Physicians. *Improving communication between doctors and patients*. London: RCP, 1997.

3 | Psychological responses to illness

SUMMARY

▶ Major health problems cause worry and distress. The degree of stress caused by an illness depends on the patient's perception of the illness rather than on the actual nature or severity of the illness.

▶ People react and cope with illness in a variety of ways. Most people, given time, develop adaptive ways to manage their illness.

▶ Although most people cope with illness, depression and anxiety disorders are twice as common in medical patients than in the general population, and are associated with significant morbidity and mortality.

▶ Depressive disorders often go unrecognised, resulting in unnecessary distress and disability.

▶ Sexual disorders are also common but often not detected by clinicians.

3.1 Introduction

Coping with illness is a dynamic process, which changes over time. People need to manage the initial emotional shock of diagnosis, assimilate information, construct an understanding of the illness and the limitations it imposes upon them, and formulate ways to cope.

Coping strategies may break down in some situations, or other factors may contribute to the development of a depressive illness or some other psychiatric condition. It is important that doctors are able to recognise and understand normal reactions to physical disease, and to detect psychiatric problems if and when they occur.

3.2 The stress associated with illness

For most patients, major health problems are perceived as stressful events. Stressful situations are typically those that are novel, unpredictable and uncontrollable, often involving change or loss. These are most intensely experienced following the diagnosis of an illness.

The stress of an illness and associated psychological responses depend more on the patient's perception of that illness than on the illness itself.[1,2] If patients perceive their illness as very threatening, or their abilities to cope with the illness as very poor, they may experience an extreme stress reaction. Anxiety and depression may be sufficiently marked to become problems in their own right. A response of denial, whilst helping to prevent extreme emotional distress in the short term, may have undesirable consequences, such as delays in seeking healthcare and non-adherence to recommended treatment. There is no clear separation between normal and abnormal psychological reactions to illness. Their significance must be judged in relation to the patient's own experience and goals, and to the likely consequences for health outcome.

The psychological care of medical patients should be based on an understanding that emotional responses and coping strategies are a normal part of illness. Patients may have different beliefs and want different types and amounts of information at different times. This makes it important to monitor the impact of previous experience and to identify the need for new information (see Table 3.1).

Table 3.1   Some useful probe questions to help doctors elicit beliefs about illness

Define context	*Sometimes it's difficult to take everything in, ...*
Elicit illness beliefs	*It would be helpful to give me an idea of what you've picked up so far, ... what you understand about your illness. Then I could perhaps fill in any gaps ... if you'd like that.*
Identify gaps	*Is there anything you're not sure of?* *or* *Is there anything you'd like me to clarify or tell you a bit more about?*
Identify concerns	*Do you have any worries or concerns about your illness?* *or* *What are the main things that concern you about your illness at the moment?*
Elicit fears	*Is there anything you're really worried about?*

3.3   Hospitalisation

Hospitalisation presents specific stresses over and above those associated with illness. Privacy, independence and social support are reduced and there is uncertainty about what will happen in hospital. High-rise buildings, lifts and long narrow corridors are unfamiliar to many. Patients are also likely to be faced with invasive and stressful medical procedures. The need for good communication and preparation from healthcare staff has already been emphasised.

A requirement of hospital admission is that patients abstain from smoking and drinking alcohol. Areas for smoking are provided in most hospitals, but these are usually off the ward, and mean that people can only smoke on an intermittent and restricted basis. If smoking, alcohol or non-prescription drugs have been used to reduce anxiety, restrictions on their use can make people more anxious and irritable than usual.

3.4   Common coping strategies

Most people have a repertoire of coping strategies which they can employ flexibly depending upon the particular circumstances.[3] The most common of these are listed in Box 3.1. Difficulties can arise if the individual has a limited range of coping responses which may themselves be affected by the illness. For example, someone who habitually deals with stress by exercising excessively, and has no other ways of reducing anxiety, will find any limitation on physical activity extremely difficult to manage.

Box 3.1   Common coping strategies

Problem-focused
  Seeking information
  Seeking practical and social support
  Learning new skills
  Actively participating in treatment
  Developing new interests or activities if previous ones are compromised by illness
  Helping others
  Becoming involved with medical charities

Emotion-focused
  Sharing feelings and concerns about illness
  Expressing anger or other distressing feelings in an appropriate way
  Acknowledging loss
  Gaining emotional support through religion
  Giving up unrealistic hopes of recovery
  Distancing (temporarily shutting off emotional worries so that one can focus on
      other tasks)

Effective communication (see Chapter 2) should enable doctors to identify particular coping strategies in different patients. Individuals who cope by gaining a sense of mastery and control over their condition will require detailed information about their illness and the treatment possibilities. However, not all individuals utilise similar strategies and others may wish to distance themselves from the minutiae of the condition. Any single coping strategy carried to an extreme is probably unhelpful.

Some other less helpful coping strategies are:

▸ Hoping and praying the condition will disappear spontaneously
▸ Denial (if it prevents the person from seeking appropriate treatment)
▸ Obsessively focusing on minute details of the disorder
▸ Seeking to blame someone (where there is no legitimate reason to do so).

3.5 Individual factors which shape people's response to illness

Personality factors influence the way people construe illness. Premorbid anxiety traits or tendencies to worry about illness can be grossly exacerbated following the development of physical symptoms. Individuals with obsessional traits who lead an ordered and controlled existence can be severely affected by physical illness, which they may feel is beyond their ability to control.

Prior experience of illness within the family can sensitise individuals to concerns about particular symptoms. People's psychological state at the time of the illness can also influence their perception of illness, eg if they happen to be depressed or suffering from anxiety when the illness develops.[4] A prior experience of trauma or a history of childhood neglect or abuse can compromise people's readiness to trust health professionals and impair their ability to cope.

If someone does not appear to be coping with illness it may be helpful to check through the questions in Box 3.2 to see if any of these personal factors are relevant.

3.6 Factors related to the illness itself

As stated above, the actual severity of the illness itself is not a major factor in determining psychological response in most cases. Certain conditions, however, are associated with high degrees of distress. Life-threatening illnesses, such as cancer, or conditions that involve the brain, are particularly difficult to come to terms with. Consideration should also be given to the potential impact of the treatment, which in some cases can be experienced as more unpleasant than the illness itself.

> **Box 3.2   Personal factors which may affect response to illness**
>
> ▶ What was this person usually like before the illness began? A worrier? Tidy or very orderly? Rather chaotic and disorganised? Aggressive/violent? Very independent?
> ▶ How were previous stresses managed?
> ▶ Is there a history of serious illness in the family?
> ▶ Was this person suffering from psychiatric illness when the physical condition began?
> ▶ Does this person have a past history of psychiatric or psychological problems?
> ▶ Is there any evidence of an extremely difficult, abusive or neglectful childhood?
> ▶ Are there any other major problems?

Acute illness

There are two patterns of acute illness to be considered from a psychological perspective:

▶ acute illness followed by complete recovery, and no long-term threat
▶ acute illness followed by disability.

If the individual is left with permanent disability, major lifestyle adjustments may be required which may be extremely difficult to achieve.

Chronic illness

Chronic illness requires a series of psychological adjustments. There are different patterns of chronic illness, including:

▶ acute relapsing with full recovery in between episodes
▶ gradual, linear decline
▶ stepwise decline with increasing disability after each discrete episode.

Some chronic illnesses, such as cancer or ischaemic heart disease, carry long-term threats to life. Others involve long-term disability.[5] With any chronic illness, the most important consideration, regarding adjustment and coping, is how the illness is perceived by the patient. Interpersonal factors and the support provided by the family and other carers have an important influence on the degree of emotional distress and disability suffered by the patient.[6,7]

Providing good care to patients with chronic physical illness should include regular review of their physical, psychological, social and spiritual needs:[8]

▶ Information about life-changing or life-threatening illnesses should be imparted with sensitivity and compassion. Doctors who do this work should have communication skills training.

▶ The assessment of chronic physical illness should include discussion of emotional, spiritual, practical and social concerns. Assessments should be repeated during the course of the illness, especially at times of relapse and during the terminal phase.

▶ An assessment should be made of carers' needs.

▶ The need for psychotherapeutic intervention or psychiatric referral should be reviewed continually.

▶ The care plan should include an appropriate response to psychosocial issues for the patient and the carer and should involve multidisciplinary teamwork.

Terminal illness

It can be very difficult for a doctor to inform a patient that the illness is terminal. Most patients, however, want to be told if their condition is terminal, and should be given as much information as they request about the illness and its probable course. One of the main roles of the doctor in this context is to ensure that the patient has a pain-free and dignified death.

Physicians can help patients adjust psychologically to their death by eliciting their concerns and responding to them in an appropriate and sympathetic manner. Religious or spiritual issues may be very important for some patients, and in all hospitals there should be access to an appropriate religious counsellor/minister. Psychological problems, including psychiatric illness, and neuro-psychiatric symptoms are very common in terminal illness.[9] It is assumed that because people are dying, depression is normal, and therefore it often goes untreated. However, the alleviation of psychological symptoms may make an important contribution to the overall experience of death for patients and their families. Good communication with the patient and family and regular assessments of their emotional needs are crucial if optimal care is to be provided.

General factors to consider in relation to managing patients with terminal illness are shown in Box 3.3.

3.7   Social context

Family members and/or friends play an important role in determining how an individual person reacts to physical symptoms. Information about illness is now

---

Box 3.3   Principles of a 'good' death (adapted from Ref 10)

Patients should:

▶ be aware that death is coming and be able to prepare themselves within the likely timescale

▶ understand what is to be expected

▶ be able to retain control over what happens

▶ be afforded dignity and privacy

▶ have control over pain relief and other symptoms

▶ have a choice and control over where death occurs

▶ have access to information and expertise of whatever kind is necessary

▶ have access to any spiritual or emotional support required

▶ have access to hospice care in any location, not only in hospital

▶ have control over who is present and who shares the end

▶ be able to issue advance directives which ensure that wishes are respected

▶ have time to say goodbye

▶ be able to leave when it is time to go and not have life prolonged pointlessly

---

available from the media, patient organisations and the worldwide web. It is difficult, however, for patients to synthesise information and make informed judgements as to the validity of their sources, so increased access to information can have both positive and deleterious effects.

Access to healthcare is determined by a variety of factors, but the most important barrier is social disadvantage. Individuals with the greatest risk factors for physical illness are the poorest in society who are also the least likely to access healthcare.

3.8   Emotional needs of carers

Demands upon the family and other carers are particularly onerous when illness is chronic and disabling. It is therefore helpful if relatives are involved in clinical management and are prepared to deal with the long-term demands that chronic illness often imposes.

There has been a lead from government for health and social services to take greater account of carers' needs.[11] This includes:

▶ encouraging more carer support services

▶ involving carers in decision-making about service provision for themselves

▶ a special grant for short-term breaks for carers.

High rates of psychological distress and depression have been found in people caring for patients with cancer[12] or stroke.[13] Medical and nursing staff therefore have a crucial role in ensuring that carers' needs are properly identified and met. This will involve close liaison with social and community services.

3.9   Adherence to medical advice and treatment

The term 'adherence' is now used in preference to 'compliance', as it suggests a more active role for patients in their healthcare. Both describe the extent to which patients engage in a range of medically recommended behaviours, including:

▶ entering into and continuing a treatment programme

▶ keeping referral and follow-up appointments

▶ taking prescribed medication correctly

▶ following recommended lifestyle changes.

Many factors can influence treatment adherence. Despite earlier claims, there is no good evidence that personality factors are involved; the same person may be adherent to one treatment but not to another. Similarly, there is no consistent evidence that socio-demographic factors, such as age or social class, are associated with adherence.

A broad distinction can be made between *unintentional* and *intentional* non-adherence. Unintentional non-adherence is primarily due to the presence of specific barriers to adherence (eg cost, access) or to communication failure, where the patient does not know or understand or has simply forgotten what has been recommended. When there are no obvious barriers and when patients are well informed about their treatment and have back-up written information, they still may not adhere to it. This is intentional non-adherence and is usually determined by patients' beliefs.[14] Patients may have negative beliefs about medicines in general which will make them less likely to adhere to any prescribed medicine. More important are the beliefs and expectations that patients have about their illness (eg whether it is seen as chronic or acute, as having serious consequences, as being amenable to cure or control) and their prescribed treatment (eg whether it is seen as effective and necessary or as having side-effects or the risk of dependence).

Although we know some of the factors which influence adherence, the evidence on the efficacy of measures designed to improve adherence is less impressive. However, the following approaches have been suggested:

▶ *Communication* – to make advice more comprehensible, concrete and memorable

▸ *Written communication* as back-up, provided it follows the recommended guidelines

▸ *General guidelines*:
  – anticipate non-adherence (assess expectations, beliefs and barriers)
  – consider patients' perspectives (their views, values and priorities)
  – establish a collaborative relationship (involvement in decision-making and planning)
  – customise treatment in the light of the above factors
  – enlist family support; involve other healthcare professionals.

3.10 Sexual problems

Sexual problems are common in the general population but are particularly widespread in general medical and surgical patients.[15,16,17] Chronic renal failure and diabetes are associated with very high rates of sexual dysfunction. Thirty-five to forty per cent of diabetic males report sexual problems.[18]

Sexual problems can be caused by:

▸ the direct effects of the condition

▸ the effects of drugs and other physical treatments

▸ psychological sequelae of the condition

▸ a co-existing psychiatric disorder (eg depression).

Sexual problems occurring in the context of physical disease should be considered as a difficulty for the couple rather than a problem specific to one person. This is important as treatment may include tasks to help the couple overcome the sexual difficulty or to adjust their usual sexual practice to accommodate changes in sexual performance caused by the illness.

Many drugs used to treat medical disorders can interfere with sexual function. It is important to note that antidepressants also affect sexual function and this should be explained to the patient if such treatment is required. Doctors rarely enquire about sexual function, and patients rarely volunteer difficulties or problems. Thus, many eminently treatable problems are not detected.[19]

Table 3.2 gives suggestions for screening questions to elicit sexual problems or difficulties. Before asking about sexual function, it is necessary to know something about the patient's social circumstances and relationships. This avoids making assumptions, for example about sexual orientation, which may lead to unnecessary embarrassment. Awareness of cultural, ethnic or religious factors is important. A detailed history is not required at this stage but it is helpful to establish what aspect of sexual function is affected so that appropriate investigation or referral can be arranged. Enquiry should proceed in a matter of fact way with sensitivity to the person's responses. It should stop if the patient appears to be embarrassed. Some clinicians may feel they require further training in this area.

For a discussion of the management of sexual problems, see Chapter 5.

Table 3.2 Asking about sexual problems

The table includes some suggestions about how to enquire about certain aspects of sexual function. All enquiries should be carried out sensitively.

STEP 1

General enquiry (establish first whether the patient has a regular sexual partner(s))	*Can I ask about the physical side of your relationship(s) … the sexual side of things?*
If in a relationship	*Are there any problems?*
If not in a relationship	*Can I ask if you have any problems with sexual function?*

STEP 2

ONLY make the following enquiries if the patient responds positively to Step 1. It is usually not appropriate to ask all of these questions. You may wish to focus on one or two areas depending upon the nature of the patient's physical complaint or disease process.

Arousal	*Do you feel interested in sex, do you get aroused? When you get aroused, do you notice a response in your body? Do you notice a wetness or lubrication in your vagina?* (women) NB: Use appropriate language according to age and background of patient.
Erection (men)	*Do you have any problems in getting an erection? Is it as firm as usual? Any problems in maintaining it? Do you get an erection in the morning?*
Ejaculation (men)	*Do you have any problems in ejaculating? Coming too early? Or not quite getting there?*
Orgasm	*Are you able to reach a climax during sex? Either during intercourse or with other kinds of sexual behaviour?*
Vaginismus (women)	*Are there any problems with actual intercourse…? Actual penetration?* (continued)

Table 3.2 (continued)

Clitoral stimulation (women)	*Can you get an orgasm if you or your partner stimulates your clitoris?*
Anal sex (heterosexual or gay relationships – only ask if relevant: establish first whether this form of penetrative sex is practised)	*There are lots of different kinds of sexual activity. Can I check whether you practise anal sex?* *If yes:* *Are there any problems with it?*
Oral sex (establish whether this form of activity is practised)	*Do you or your partner use oral ways of stimulating each other during sex and getting an orgasm?* *If yes:* *Are there any problems or difficulties?*
Other types of sexual activity	*Are there any other problems about the sexual side of things that we haven't mentioned that you'd like to discuss?*

3.11 Psychiatric disorders in the general hospital setting

Although most people develop adaptive ways to manage their illness, a small minority may develop psychiatric illness which requires treatment. It is sometimes difficult for physicians to distinguish between 'normal' distress and psychiatric disorder. In many people, a change in mood is brief in duration and resolves when the physical illness improves. The mood change should then be regarded as an adjustment disorder rather than a psychiatric disorder requiring active treatment. The latter should be considered either when a change of mood is persistent, extreme or disabling or when the symptoms are unusual or bizarre (psychotic symptoms). The most common psychiatric disorders in the medically ill are depressive and anxiety disorders. Psychotic disorders are relatively rare, but can evoke disquiet in medical and nursing staff if patients with these problems have to be nursed in a general medical setting.

There are no diagnostic tests for psychiatric disorders. Diagnosis continues to be determined by clinical assessment conducted by an experienced psychiatrist. Structured diagnostic systems have been developed to improve consistency. The two most widely used are the American DSM-IV (*Diagnostic and Statistical Manual of Mental Disorders*, 4th edn)[20] and the World Health Organisation's *International Classification of Diseases*.[21] The manuals are most useful for research purposes where diagnostic consistency is a prerequisite. In clinical practice they provide a useful framework but rigid adherence can be unhelpful, particularly in relation to psychiatric conditions which occur in the context of physical disorder. For example, a diabetic patient with a relatively mild eating disorder, which does not fulfil the criteria for bulimia nervosa, may nevertheless have severe problems with diabetic control with potentially serious long-term consequences.

3.12 Depressive disorders in the medically ill

Major depression is twice as common in medical patients in general hospitals as in the general population. It is associated with significant morbidity and mortality. However, depressive disorders are inadequately detected and treated by hospital doctors and general practitioners. As well as alleviating the severe distress caused to the patient, there are several other important reasons for treating depression in the medical setting:

Depressed patients are more likely than non-depressed patients to:

- commit suicide[22,23,24]
- spend more time in hospital and have more outpatient visits[25]
- have greater disability[26]
- have a poorer quality of life.[25,27]

Characteristics of depression

All depressive disorders are characterised by a lowering of mood which is severe and persistent. Symptoms can be divided into three main areas: mood and motivation, cognitive changes and biological features (see Box 3.4).

Detection of depression

Detection of depression in the medically ill can be difficult for two reasons. First, staff may regard the patient's distress as a normal reaction to physical illness. They may imagine themselves facing similar trauma, but fail to understand that most individuals develop ways of coping with illness if they are given support and time to adjust. Second, the common somatic symptoms of depression (eg weight loss, anorexia, tiredness) are often due to the medical illness, so the normal symptom pattern cannot be relied upon to a make a definitive diagnosis. Positive answers to the following questions should raise awareness of the possibility of depression:

▶ Does the person's distress appear to be very severe?

▶ Is the mood change persistent? (ie lasting more than two weeks)

Box 3.4   Depressive symptoms

Mood and motivation symptoms
   Persistently lowered mood (may be worse in the morning)
   Diminished interest or pleasure in almost all activities (anhedonia)
   Social withdrawal
   Loss of energy
   Poor concentration

Cognitive changes
   Depressive ideation: feelings of guilt, worthlessness, self-blame
   Suicidal thoughts
   Hopelessness

Biological symptoms
   Poor appetite, loss of enjoyment of food
   Significant weight loss when not dieting
   Sleep disturbance most days (either initial insomnia or early morning waking)
   Retardation or agitation
   Decreased sex drive

Symptoms must be persistent and present for at least two weeks.

▶ Is there evidence of a failure to adjust to the illness?

▶ Is the person expressing suicidal ideas?

▶ Is the person's physical function poorer than expected?

▶ Is the person's recovery from illness slower than expected, or is rehabilitation difficult?

▶ Is there poor social interaction? (eg the patient does not respond to relatives visiting, staff or other patients on the ward)

Particular attention should be given to the affective and cognitive symptoms of depression (see Box 3.4). Suicidal feelings should always be taken seriously, and are very rarely a normal reaction to physical illness. Some patients with terminal

---

Box 3.5   Simple questions to elicit alcohol use in the context of depression

Do you ever have a drink to relieve stress or cheer yourself up?
Have you been drinking more than usual?
Roughly how much have you been drinking?

illness may decide they wish to die, but there is usually evidence of careful and thoughtful deliberation over a period of months.

If there is a positive response to the initial screen, specific questions to elicit affective and cognitive symptoms of depression can be used (see Table 3.3). Alcohol use may increase as a consequence of depression, which may further lower mood, and simple questions may be asked to elicit alcohol use (see Box 3.5). For further information about screening for alcohol problems, see Chapter 7.

Table 3.3 Depression: asking about emotional and cognitive symptoms

Symptom	Question
Low mood	*How are you feeling in your spirits, in your mood?*
Tearfulness	*Do you find yourself in tears?* or *Are you any more weepy than normal?*
Anhedonia	*Do you cheer up sometimes, even though you're in hospital? Do you enjoy the things you used to?*
Loss of interest	*Are you able to keep interests going?*
Poor concentration	*How is your concentration? Can you read the paper or watch TV and take it in?*
Irritability	*Are you more snappy than usual?*
Panic attacks	*Do you get panicky at all?*
Diurnal variation of mood	*Is your mood worse at any particular time of day?* *How do you feel when you first wake up?*
Guilt, self-blame	*Do you find yourself blaming yourself or regretting things?* *Do you ever feel a burden to others?*
Worthlessness, low self-esteem	*How do you view yourself, in comparison with others?* *Do you ever feel very unsure of yourself inside or feel you have little to offer compared with others?*
Pessimism, hopelessness	*How do you see the future?*
Thoughts of dying	Step 1: *Are there ever times when you feel you just want to go to sleep and never wake up?*
Suicidal ideation	If yes to Step 1, Step 2: *Have you thought of harming yourself or taking your own life?*

Depression associated with particular physical disorders or treatment

The prevalence of depression is particularly high in certain physical conditions or groups of patients. These include:

▶ illnesses which affect the brain, eg stroke, Parkinson's disease, multiple sclerosis

▶ life-threatening disorders, eg cancer, HIV/AIDS

▶ chronic, painful, disabling illnesses which impede self-care, eg rheumatoid arthritis

▶ unpleasant treatments, eg chemotherapy

▶ chronic illness in old age.

For discussion of treatments of depression, see Chapter 5.

3.13 Anxiety states in the medically ill

Normal worry provides an important function in motivating people to solve problems. Excessive worry is disabling, counterproductive and uncontrollable. Anxiety disorders are characterised by excessive or problematic worrying, as a consequence of which individuals become distressed or dysfunctional. The main features of each disorder are summarised in Table 3.4. There is much overlap between these conditions, and they often coexist with depression.

Pure anxiety states are much less common than depression in the medically ill, but are more likely to be recognised by hospital staff. Patients with ischaemic heart disease may present with episodes of panic and chest pain, which are difficult to distinguish clinically from angina. Individuals with type I diabetes may develop a phobic reaction to injecting themselves with insulin (needle phobia). Anxiety is common following cortical lesions in stroke.

Acute injury as a consequence of a road traffic accident or assault is associated with high levels of anxiety. Flashbacks or vivid dreams are common and should not be regarded as pathological in the immediate aftermath of a severe trauma. These experiences usually subside within six to eight weeks. Post-traumatic stress disorder and other anxiety states such as phobic anxiety disorder occur in up to one-third of cases.[28] Routine psychological debriefing following the trauma is not beneficial[29] and may even be harmful for some patients.[30,31] Those with a prior history of psychiatric illness, psychiatric morbidity at the time of the acute stressor, or a particularly severe response to the trauma should be monitored closely, as they are at greater risk of developing persistent problems.

Table 3.4 The main features of anxiety disorders

Type of disorder	Main features
Panic disorder	Recurrent and unexpected panic attacks, with or without anxiety between attacks
Agoraphobia	Fear and avoidance of being in public places or enclosed situations from which escape may be difficult
Generalised anxiety disorder	Excessive anxiety and worry not linked to specific objects or situations
Specific phobia	Abnormal fear and avoidance of specific objects or situations, eg blood, needles
Social phobia	Persistent fear and avoidance of social situations in which embarrassment may occur
Obsessional compulsive disorder	Persistent, intrusive, unwanted thoughts or images that are difficult to resist, and are recognised by the person as their own. Associated ritualistic behaviour may develop
Post-traumatic stress disorder	Intrusive, recurrent thoughts or images of a traumatic experience, with avoidance of stimuli associated with the trauma, and generalised background anxiety

3.14 Psychosis

Schizophrenia is the commonest reason for admission to a psychiatric inpatient unit, but it is relatively rare in the general hospital setting. Patients with schizophrenia or bipolar affective disorder may be admitted to the general hospital following a serious episode of self-harm and they should receive prompt psychiatric assessment.

Brief psychotic states can be produced by various drugs, including steroids and anti-parkinsonian agents. Other psychotic states often develop in the context of an underlying delirium and remit once the cause is treated. Organic conditions are discussed in more detail in Chapter 8. Occasionally, patients develop acute paranoid states in clear consciousness as a reaction to being placed in fearful or unusual surroundings, particularly coronary care or intensive treatment units. The paranoid delusions often involve medical and nursing staff.

3.15 Other psychiatric conditions

Other common psychiatric conditions in the medical setting, including deliberate self-harm, alcohol problems and delirium, are discussed in Chapters 6, 7 and 8.

References

1 Leventhal H, Leventhal EA, Schaefer PM. Vigilant coping and health behaviour. In Ory MG, Abeles RP, Lipman PD (eds) *Aging, health, and behavior.* Thousand Oaks, CA: Sage Publications, 1992:109–40.

2 Scharloo M, Kaptein AA, Weinman J, Hazes JM *et al.* Illness perceptions, coping and functioning in patients with rheumatoid arthritis, chronic obstructive pulmonary disease and psoriasis. *J Psychosom Res* 1998;**44**(5):573–85.

3 Weinman J. Coping with illness and handicap. In Weinman J (ed) *An outline of psychology as applied to medicine.* London: Butterworth-Heinemann, 1987:190–207.

4 Nickel R, Wunsch A, Egle UT, Lohse AW, Otto G. The relevance of anxiety, depression, and coping in patients after liver transplantation. *Liver Transpl* 2002;**8**(1):63–71.

5 Mayou R. The relationship between physical illness and psychiatric pathology. In House A, Mayou R, Mallinson C (eds) *Psychiatric aspects of disease.* London: Royal College of Physicians and Royal College of Psychiatrists, 1995:3–7.

6 Singer JE, Lord D. The role of social support in coping with chronic or life threatening illness. In Baum A, Singer JE, Taylor S (eds) *Handbook of psychology and health,* vol IV. Hillsdale, NJ: Erlbaum, 1984.

7 MacMahon KM, Lip GY. Psychological factors in heart failure: a review of the literature. *Arch Intern Med* 2002;**162**(5):509–16.

8 McIllmurray MB, Thomas C, Francis B, Morris S *et al.* The psychosocial needs of cancer patients: findings from an observational study. *Eur J Cancer* 2001;**10**:261–9.

9 Breibart W, Bruera E, Chochinov H, Lynch M. Neuropsychiatric syndromes and psychological symptoms in patients with advanced cancer. *J Pain Symptom Manage* 1995;**10**:131–41.

10 Age Concern. *The future of health and care of older people: the best is yet to come.* London: Age Concern, 1999.

11 Department of Health. *Caring about cancers: a national strategy for carers.* London: DH, 1999.

12 Krishnasamy M, Wilkie E, Haviland J. Lung cancer health care needs assessment: patients' and informal carers' responses to a national mail questionnaire survey. *Palliat Med* 2001;**15**(3):213–27.

13 Sinnakaruppan I, Williams DM. Family carers and the adult head-injured: a critical review of carers' needs. *Brain Injury* 2001;**15**(8):653–72.

14 Horne R, Weinman J. Patients' beliefs about prescribed medicines and their role in adherence to treatment in chronic physical illness. *J Psychosom Res* 1999;**47**(6): 555–67.

15 Nazareth I, Lewin J, King M. Sexual dysfunction after treatment for testicular cancer: a systematic review. *J Psychosom Res* 2001;**51**(6):735–43.

16 Sipski ML. Sexual function in women with neurologic disorders. *Phys Med Rehabil Clin N America* 2001;**12**(1):79–90.

17 Incrocci L, Slob AK, Levendag PC. Sexual dysfunction after radiotherapy for prostate cancer: a review. *Inl J Radiat Oncol Biol Phys* 2002;**52**(3):681–93.

18   Guay AT. Sexual dysfunction in the diabetic patient. *Int J Impotence Res* 2001; 13(Suppl 5):S47–50,

19   Burchardt M, Burchardt T, Anastasiadis AG, Kiss AJ *et al*. Sexual dysfunction is common and overlooked in female patients with hypertension *J Sex Marit Ther* 2002;28(1):17–26.

20   American Psychiatric Association. *Diagnostic and statistical manual of mental disorders*, 4th edn (DSM-IV). Washington DC: APA, 1994.

21   World Health Organization. *International classification of diseases*, 10th edn (ICD-10). Geneva: WHO, 1992.

22   Roose SP, Dalack GW, Woodring S. Death, depression, and heart disease. *J Clin Psychiatry* 1991;52(Suppl):34–9.

23   Frasure-Smith N, Lesperance F, Talajic M. Depression following myocardial infarction: impact on 6-month survival. *JAMA* 1993;270:1819–25.

24   Hoyer EH, Mortensen PB, Olesen AV. Mortality and causes of death in a total national sample of patients with affective disorders admitted for the first time between 1973 and 1993. *Br J Psychiat* 2000;176:76–82.

25   Koenig HG, Kuchibhatla M. Use of health services by hospitalized medically ill depressed elderly patients. *Am J Psychiat* 1998;155(7):871–7.

26   Pohjasvaara T, Vataja R, Leppavuori A, Kaste M, Erkinjuntti T. Depression is an independent predictor of poor long-term functional outcome post-stroke. *Eur J Neurol* 2001;8(4):315–9.

27   Robinson-Smith G, Johnston MV. Allen J. Self-care, self-efficacy, quality of life, and depression after stroke. *Arch Phys Med Rehabil* 2000;81(4):460–4.

28   Mayou R, Bryant B. Outcome in consecutive emergency department attenders following a road traffic accident. *Br J Psychiat* 2001;179:528–34.

29   Wessely S, Rose S, Bisson J. A systematic review of brief psychological interventions ('debriefing') for the treatment of immediate trauma-related symptoms and the prevention of post traumatic stress disorder. Cochrane Collaboration. *Cochrane Library*, Issue 4. Oxford: Update Software, 1999.

30   Kenardy JA, Webster RA, Lewin TJ, Carr VJ *et al*. Stress debriefing and patterns of recovery following a natural disaster. *J Trauma Stress* 1996;9:37–49.

31   Bisson J, Jenkins P, Alexander J, Bannister C. Randomised controlled trial of psychological debriefing for victims of acute burn trauma. *Br J Psychiat* 1997;171:78–81.

Further reading

Baum A, Newman S, Weinman J, West R, McManus C (eds) *Cambridge handbook of psychology, health and medicine*. New York, NY: Cambridge University Press, 1997.

Guthrie E, Creed F (eds). *Seminars in liaison psychiatry*. London: Gaskell/Royal College of Psychiatrists, 1996.

House A, Mayou R, Mallinson C (eds).*Psychiatric aspects of physical disease*. London: Royal College of Physicians and Royal College of Psychiatrists, 1995.

Sutor B, Rummans TA, Jowsey SG, Krahn LE *et al*. Major depression in medically ill patients. *Mayo Clin Proc* 1998;73(4):329–37.

Websites

www.nimh.nih.gov/publicat/index.cfm#disinfo
    Useful website which gives authoritative information regarding specific psychiatric disorders.

www.cancerbacup.org.uk/info/depress/depress-15.htm
  Website for cancer sufferers with depression. Provides very good, simple advice.
www.rcpsych.ac.uk
  Website of the Royal College of Psychiatrists. Provides helpful advice for patients and
  professionals.

4 | Medically unexplained symptoms

SUMMARY

▶ The current management and help offered to patients with medically unexplained symptoms is largely inadequate.

▶ The National Service Framework on Mental Health does not include reference to such patients or consider the psychological needs of such patients in the general hospital setting. Therefore, funding for psychological services for patients with medically unexplained symptoms is unlikely to come from mental health services.

▶ Patients with severe or chronic medically unexplained symptoms are costly to the health service and a financial burden to society. There is good evidence that patients with mild disorders of recent onset respond to reassurance and explanation. Those with moderate disorders usually respond to brief psychological interventions or psychotropic treatment.

▶ Patients with more chronic and severe conditions may benefit from more intensive psychological management or treatment in a specific medical rehabilitation unit.

▶ Services for patients with medically unexplained symptoms need to be developed if adequate treatment and management are to be provided.

4.1   Introduction

Some patients present with physical symptoms for which there is no obvious underlying organic cause, or which are disproportionate to underlying detectable pathology. In many cases, but not all, the presentation is associated with underlying psychiatric disorder. Such conditions are known by a variety of different terms, the current favourite being 'medically unexplained symptoms', as this does not imply any aetiological cause.

These conditions are poorly understood, but it is unhelpful to think of them in either purely physical or psychiatric terms. The experience of any physical or emotional state in the body is obviously mediated by an underlying physiological process, so the term 'medically unexplained' is a misnomer. A more helpful approach may to be to consider the relative contribution of physiological, psychological and behavioural factors in a particular condition.

4.2   Terminology

Some of the terms used in relation to medically unexplained conditions are confusing and tend to be used indiscriminately. Brief definitions for the different terms are provided in Table 4.1.

Although formal definitions exist for these various disorders, in reality patients often do not fit neatly into one category or another. There is a spectrum of conditions in which

▶ 'medically unexplained' symptoms may be superimposed on a background of greater or lesser degrees of identifiable organic pathology

▶ patients have varying degrees of insight or acknowledgement that a proportion of their symptoms are related to psychological factors

▶ patients may demonstrate a range of different behaviours and beliefs which contribute to their overall condition.

'Abnormal illness behaviour' describes a behavioural response to a physical condition which is out of proportion to the underlying problem. Contributory factors include illness beliefs (for example that bed-rest will cure the problem) or secondary gains (such as increased attention from friends and family, or financial reward in the form of sickness benefits). It is part of the normal human condition to exaggerate. We may or may not have insight into this behaviour, or be prepared to admit to it. Families may be unwittingly drawn into an excessively caring role or may find themselves colluding with the dependent behaviour in the belief that they are helping. The collection of visible props such as neck collars, wrist splints and walking aids is sometimes adopted as a way of coping. It engenders a solicitous response from others, but emphasises the physical nature of the problem since this may be perceived as more acceptable than demonstrating signs of psychological distress.

In defining 'organic pathology' it is important to remember that medical investigations are fairly crude and generally set at a level sensitive enough only to identify clinically important pathology. The absence of demonstrable pathology, therefore, does not always exclude its presence. The purpose of identifying overlying symptoms or behaviours is not to imply that the condition is any the less important, but simply that different management strategies may be required. Physical symptoms are unlikely to resolve unless the psychological factors are actively addressed. It is important, therefore, that the physician takes a holistic view and teases out these various different components in order to direct treatment appropriately. This will avoid excessive use of medical intervention, with all its accompanying risks, for problems which are not likely to be responsive to that approach alone.

Table 4.1 Terminology

Somatoform disorders

Collective term given to a series of psychiatric diagnoses in which the principal symptomatic concern is a preoccupation with physical symptoms.
Symptoms:
▶ cause significant distress and/or impairment
▶ are disproportionate to underlying organic disease
▶ are not intentionally produced or feigned
▶ are not better accounted for by other psychiatric conditions
▶ are precipitated and maintained by psychological factors

Somatisation disorder:	At least 8 different somatic symptoms, in different sites of the body with no demonstrable organic findings, and positive evidence that they are linked to psychological factors
Psychogenic pain disorder:	Preoccupation with pain in absence of physical explanation
Body dysmorphic disorder:	Excessive concern about a trivial or non-existent bodily deformity
Conversion disorder:	Symptom or deficit affecting voluntary motor or sensory function that suggests a neurological condition, but cannot be explained by organic causes
Hypochondriasis:	Preoccupation with the fear or belief that one has a serious disease. Rarely responds to reassurance or explanation

Functional somatic syndromes

Collective term used to describe medically unexplained symptom clusters. Different functional syndromes have been described according to the different bodily systems and medical specialties. Common examples include:

Gastroenterology	Irritable bowel syndrome; functional dyspepsia
Neurology	Chronic fatigue syndrome
Cardiology	Atypical chest pain; hyperventilation
Urology	Irritable bladder
Rheumatology	Fibromyalgia; repetitive strain injury
Clinical immunology	Multiple chemical sensitivity syndrome
Gynaecology	Chronic pelvic pain
Orthopaedics	Chronic back pain

Feigned disorders

Factitious disorder:	Physical or psychological symptoms which are intentionally produced or feigned in order to assume the sick role, in the absence of obvious external reasons for doing so
Malingering:	Intentional production or feigning of symptoms, with underlying external motivator, eg a wish for compensation or avoidance of prison

4.3   Prevalence

Medically unexplained symptoms are relatively common in community samples,[1] but the extreme forms, which warrant classification as psychiatric disorders, are relatively rare.[2]

General practitioners (GPs) see large numbers of patients with somatisation.[3,4] Approximately one-quarter of all patients who seek help from their GP do so because of physical symptoms which cannot be explained by underlying organic disease, but are related to psychological distress.

In the general hospital setting, medically unexplained symptoms are common in outpatient clinics but rarer in the inpatient setting. Approximately 40–50% of patients in hospital outpatient clinics have unexplained medical symptoms.[5] The more somatic symptoms people report, the greater the likelihood of associated mental illness, regardless of the nature of the symptoms.[6]

4.4   Aetiology

Recognised aetiological factors in medically unexplained symptoms include:

▶ *Childhood experience of illness* – particularly when coupled with lack of parental care, either because of the loss of a parent through death, or because of a physically or sexually abusive relationship.[7,8] Children whose emotional needs are neglected by their parents may learn that physical illness elicits care and attention, either from their parents or others, which they would not receive otherwise.

▶ *Lack of social support and confiding relationships* – this may increase physiological arousal and preoccupation with somatic symptoms.

▶ *A tendency to worry about illness* and selectively attend to bodily symptoms – this can increase anxiety, and encourage checking behaviours, which reinforce illness beliefs.[9]

▶ *Family reinforcement* of the patient's belief that he is ill, eg by over-solicitous care, or by offering 'helpful' advice.

▶ *Isolated older people* who feel their medical needs are unrecognised may realise that physical symptoms trigger support and help.

▶ *Iatrogenic causes* which result from the medicalisation of symptoms[10] including:
  – overinvestigation and inappropriate treatment which reinforces the patient's illness beliefs
  – failure to provide a clear explanation for symptoms and appropriate

reassurance, resulting in uncertainty and increased anxiety in the patient

– failure to recognise and treat important emotional factors underlying the symptom presentation.

4.5   Consequences of failure to manage medically unexplained symptoms

The long-term consequences of failures in the management of medically unexplained symptoms can result in a variety of deleterious effects which are listed in Box 4.1.

Box 4.1   Long-term consequences of failure to manage medically unexplained symptoms

Physical consequences for the patient

▶ prescribed drug misuse with dependence

▶ untreated psychiatric illness[11]

▶ iatrogenic illness: eg polysurgery

Social consequences for the patient and his/her family

▶ disability and loss of earnings

▶ incapacity benefit[12]

▶ poor social functioning and quality of life[13]

▶ secondary impact on family and social network

▶ long-term institutional care for older adults

Consequences for the NHS

▶ unnecessary and expensive investigations[14]

▶ repeated admissions to hospital[15]

▶ frequent attendance at outpatient clinics

4.6   Factitious disorders and malingering

▶ *Factitious disorders* are characterised by 'physical or psychological symptoms which are intentionally produced or feigned in order to assume the sick role'.[16] Central to the definition must be an absence of other forms of external incentives for the condition. These disorders are relatively uncommon but probably underdiagnosed.

▶ *Malingering* also involves the intentional production or feigning of symptoms, but there is an underlying external motivator, such as a wish for compensation or avoidance of prison.

Most of the literature consists of case descriptions of different presentations in which patients have managed to fabricate illness – some of which are ingenious and require detailed medical knowledge – but they probably represent the extreme end of the spectrum. Given the intentional nature of the condition, the majority of true malingerers are often reluctant to accept psychological or psychiatric help.[17] Challenging them directly is likely to be unhelpful and may encourage them to go elsewhere, sometimes assuming a different name.

In reality, it is often extremely difficult to establish (a) that symptoms have been intentionally fabricated, and (b) if they have, the motivation for the dissimulating behaviour. In cases of medico-legal compensation or of suspected Munchausen's syndrome by proxy, where another party is at risk, the fabrication of symptoms can be established using covert surveillance. Such methods, however, have ethical implications and are impractical in most clinical settings. In a busy general medical ward it is impossible to monitor patients' behaviour in the detail required to confirm fabrication. This often makes the management of such cases extremely difficult, and can result in an escalation of the behaviour, or a complete breakdown in the relationship between staff and patient.

Where staff suspect that components of illness behaviour are 'volitional' (that is, intentionally produced or exaggerated), it is appropriate to document that behaviour as carefully as possible, together with the reasons for suspecting its volitional nature and any identified external motivation or gain. A recognised pattern of behaviour may thus be identified.

4.7   Management of patients with medically unexplained symptoms

General measures

Many health professionals shy away from discussing the psychological aspects of disease. This may result from uncertainty about the boundaries between organic disease and psychological problems, as described above. Alternatively, they may believe that they are reassuring the patient by stating baldly that the symptoms are not due to organic disease. Unfortunately, patients may then feel they are being told that there is nothing wrong and are left either believing that the physician has not understood their symptoms or wondering whether they have some sinister disease that has not been diagnosed. A suggested approach is outlined in Box 4.2.

> **Box 4.2   A suggested approach for addressing medically unexplained symptoms**
>
> During the initial assessment, carry out a **brief psychosocial assessment:**
>
> ▸ Do not wait until all the medical investigations have been completed and are normal, before enquiring about psychological factors. Do this in a matter-of-fact way.
>
> ▸ Check for problems with mood, current life stressors, previous psychiatric illness and childhood adversity.
>
> ▸ Elicit the patient's concerns and beliefs about his/her condition.
>
> **Provide an explanation** for the symptoms, in terms that the patient can understand:
>
> ▸ This explanation should encompass the physical, psychological and behavioural factors involved, and how they might be addressed.
>
> ▸ Analogies with normal physiological reactions to stress may help patients and relatives to understand and accept the explanation.
>
> **Reassurance** should be based firmly on a knowledge of the patient's particular worries.

Patients with medically unexplained symptoms who receive clear information and are provided with strategies to cope, feel empowered[18] and are more likely to accept advice and reassurance.

Psychological or drug treatments

If patients do not respond to reassurance and their symptoms continue to cause distress, referral for psychological treatment should be considered. This may be to a liaison psychiatry service or clinical or health psychology services.

Antidepressants may be helpful (see Chapter 5). However, they should be used only if psychological screening demonstrates significant depressive symptoms and should be prescribed only after an adequate explanation of their nature and purpose has been given.

Brief psychological treatments, including cognitive behavioural therapy, psychodynamic interpersonal therapy and counselling (see Chapter 5), have been shown to be effective for certain functional somatic syndromes. Most treatments are conducted on an outpatient basis and are suitable for patients with mild to moderate symptoms or symptoms of less than two years duration. Hypnosis may also be effective, although it is not widely available.

4.8   Management of chronic and severe medically unexplained symptoms

For most patients with severe unexplained symptoms, management of their symptoms, rather than attempts to cure, is the most appropriate form of care. In today's NHS there is great pressure to treat and discharge patients as soon as possible. Unfortunately, the lesser the organic component of disease, the less successful this approach becomes. Patients with chronic or multiple medically unexplained symptoms pose a significant challenge in the context of a busy medical service. These patients exist in almost every specialty area of medicine and are frequently referred to as 'fat-file' or 'heart-sink' patients after the tell-tale clues or the feelings engendered in the doctor when such a patient enters the consulting room. These terms themselves indicate the need for a clear management strategy on the part of the staff who care for them. Doctors who try to achieve great changes with such patients are often disappointed. A conservative management policy, which reduces both disability and the use of expensive investigation, is preferable.

Assessment

Aims

The key to appropriate management is a detailed assessment which elicits the various components contributing to the patient's presentation. The main aims of the assessment are to:

▶ establish the nature and extent of any underlying pathology
▶ determine the nature and extent of the overlying non-organic component
▶ identify any treatable psychological component
▶ identify factors which help to maintain the symptoms
▶ ascertain the extent of the patient's motivation for change.

Life-symptom chart

There is often a previous history of nonspecific symptoms. The GP notes should be requested and one of the team should construct a summary chart of the patient's previous contact with services (see Table 4.2). Although this takes a considerable amount of time to prepare, it is of great value. The development of the patient's symptoms can be tracked through the GP notes, and the pattern of treatment-seeking established. The hospital medical notes usually contain only a fraction of the patient's symptomatic and consultation history.

History, psychosocial assessment, examination and review

A careful history should be taken along with a brief psychosocial assessment (Box 4.2), a detailed examination and a review of previous investigations, based

Bass C, Peveler R, House A. Somatoform disorders: severe psychiatric illnesses neglected by psychiatrists. *Br J Psychiat* 2001;**179**:11–14.

Halligan P, Bass C, Marshall JC (eds). *Contemporary approaches to the study of hysteria: clinical and theoretical perspectives.* Oxford: Oxford University Press, 2001.

5 | Management of psychological problems

SUMMARY

▶ Relatives and carers should be involved in treatment at various stages if the patient consents.

▶ Counselling and specific psychological treatments are effective in alleviating psychological symptoms.

▶ Medication has an important role in treating anxiety and depression. Antidepressants are probably under-prescribed in the medically ill.

▶ Referral to a psychiatrist or psychologist is required for a minority of patients with psychological symptoms.

▶ Many sexual problems respond to counselling or pharmacological treatment.

5.1 Prevention: giving adequate information in advance

As with many areas of medicine, prevention is better than cure. Good communication is essential if the psychological problems associated with illness are to be minimised (see Chapter 2). Adequate information and preparation given in advance of a planned medical or surgical procedure reduce anxiety and pain, and speed recovery.[1]

5.2 Involving patients and their families

Involving patients and their families is a critical part of management. The clinician needs to spend time explaining the illness and its treatment, and offering support as necessary. Patients frequently need to hear information a number of times before they remember and understand what they have been told. Information leaflets are useful supplements but should not replace verbal communication. Patients can also derive considerable support from members of a peer group with similar problems.

Patients need to be aware that physical illness often leads to a change in circumstances which engenders a normal psychological reaction. In most cases, this mood change is transient, resolving when the physical illness improves or when the patient learns to adjust to persisting disability.

5.3   Support for families and carers

Illness and disability affect whole families, not just individuals. Relatives and carers require support in their own right but they should only be involved in discussions of treatment if the patient consents. Solicitous caring for the individual through an acute illness may become ingrained so that families can become overprotective, and unwittingly contribute to the patient's continuing dependence and disability, even after physical improvement has occurred.

Relatives may need permission or even encouragement to withdraw and allow the patient to acquire more independence. This is facilitated if they are given information to help them understand the true limitations that the patient faces. Involvement in therapy sessions may be appropriate in this context. Peer group support for carers is also helpful.

5.4   General support and counselling

Having given patients an explanation for their symptoms, the first line of management is usually to offer authoritative reassurance that treatment is available and that recovery or improvement are anticipated. It is also helpful to offer advice that will allow patients to take some responsibility for managing their own symptoms while deriving support from health professionals. This includes:

▸ Simple advice and problem-solving – helping them to address the practical issues which can otherwise weigh them down. Interdisciplinary teamwork is essential to link the patient with appropriate networks of statutory and voluntary support. Specialist nurses may be particularly important in this respect. They have become essential members of multidisciplinary teams in several specialties including diabetic medicine, oncology and HIV/AIDS. Primary healthcare services should also be involved.

▸ Counselling services – these should be used when appropriate once patients have been assessed to ensure that they do not have a serious psychological disorder that requires specific treatment. Problem-focused counselling is effective. A widely used approach proceeds through three stages:

1 Problem exploration and clarification

2 Goal-setting

3 Facilitating action.

▶ Specific techniques, such as relaxation and breathing exercises – these may help prevent exacerbation of symptoms and reduce some of the unwanted physiological consequences of anxiety such as tremor, paraesthesia, and muscle tension.

5.5   Self-help: spiritual and cultural support

In a medical model of care it is easy to forget the benefit that patients and their families derive from taking positive steps to help themselves, and from sharing their experiences with others who are coping with similar adversity. Staff should consider what forms of cultural or spiritual support might be available. This is particularly important when the patient has different religious and cultural beliefs from the doctor responsible for treatment. Hospital chaplains have taken on an extended role and may be helpful not only in exploring patients' beliefs and cultural backgrounds, but also in providing details of local spiritual and cultural support. Information and contact details about suitable self-help groups should also be provided.

5.6   Drug treatments suitable for use by the physician

Treatment for anxiety and panic attacks

Certain drugs may be helpful when used for a short duration:

▶ Brief treatment with low-dose benzodiazepines may be appropriate for inpatients to help with periods of insomnia or stress of limited duration, but it is essential that these drugs be stopped before discharge because of the risk of dependence. Their use for outpatients must also be limited. Hospital doctors should confer with the patient's GP before starting such medication, which should be stopped within a period of three weeks.

▶ Certain somatic symptoms of anxiety, eg palpitations and tremor, respond well to beta-blockers. A small dose of a non-selective agent, eg 10–20 mg propranolol, may be more effective than selective agents such as atenolol.

▶ Antidepressants (see below) are effective for panic attacks and post-traumatic stress disorder.

Treatment for depression

Patients with significant depression should be considered for antidepressant therapy, especially when their mood disorder is persistent and hindering recovery or rehabilitation. Before starting such treatment, patients should be given adequate information about their condition and the role of antidepressants, as listed in Box 5.1.

> **Box 5.1 Patient information on antidepressants**
>
> **Before starting antidepressants, patients should be aware:**
> - of the biochemical basis for depression, and that mood is maintained by a balance of biochemical factors within the brain, which can be altered as a direct physiological consequence of disease
> - that modern treatments for depression restore the balance of chemistry within the brain towards normal, thus enabling patients to cope with their situation in a more normal state of mood
> - that the effect may take 2–4 weeks to become apparent, and that treatment needs to be continued regularly for at least 6 months to achieve full effect and prevent relapse. In patients who repeatedly relapse, long-term maintenance medication is recommended
> - of the possible side-effects of the medication which has been prescribed for them

Antidepressant drugs are probably underprescribed in medically ill patients. Several factors account for this:
- the depression is not recognised
- depression is regarded as a normal, understandable response
- doctors fear the side effects of medication on the underlying illness
- drug interactions are not known.

Once a decision to treat has been agreed, the choice of drug will depend to a large extent on known side-effects and potential interactions with other drugs. The two main drug groups remain the tricyclics and the selective serotonin reuptake inhibitors (SSRIs). Of the other older antidepressants, the monoamine oxidase inhibitors (MAOIs) are indicated for atypical depression when the low mood is accompanied by weight gain, hypersomnia and profound fatigue. They have the major disadvantage of interacting with various drugs and tyramine-containing foods, with the risk of producing a potentially fatal hypertensive crisis. The risk is considerably reduced with the reversible MAOI, moclobemide.

A *Cochrane Review* has specifically examined the efficacy of antidepressants in patients with medical illness.[2] On the evidence available from 18 controlled studies the following conclusions could be drawn:
- Antidepressants brought about significantly greater reduction in depression than either placebo or no treatment in patients with a wide range of illnesses.

▶ Approximately four patients would need to be treated to produce one recovery from depression which would not have occurred had they been given placebo.

▶ Antidepressants seemed reasonably acceptable to patients.

▶ There was a trend towards tricyclics being more effective than SSRIs.

▶ Tricyclics were associated with a higher drop-out rate.

SSRIs have replaced tricyclics as the drugs of first choice in depression because of their better side-effect profile and their greater safety in overdose. These factors are particularly important in the medically ill. Five SSRIs are currently available – fluoxetine, fluvoxamine, paroxetine, sertraline and citalopram. There are important pharmacokinetic differences between them,[3] notably in their ability to inhibit hepatic cytochrome P450 isoenzymes which are responsible for the metabolism of many drugs. *In vitro* studies suggest that citalopram and sertraline are least likely to inhibit these isoenzymes and are therefore least likely to cause interactions with other drugs. The choice of drug should be matched to the patient's individual needs as far as possible,[4] depending on the effect and tolerability of previous treatment with an SSRI, whether sedation is required and the risks of interactions.[3] Some patients experience a withdrawal syndrome when stopping SSRIs so the dose of the drugs must always be reduced gradually.

Newer antidepressants

Four antidepressants – venlafaxine, nefazodone, mirtazapine and reboxetine – have been introduced since the SSRIs were developed. They have significantly different pharmacological properties and are claimed to have greater specificity, equivalent or better efficacy and fewer side effects than the earlier classes of antidepressants.[5] Sexual dysfunction, a common problem with SSRIs, is rare with nefazodone, mirtazapine and reboxetine which are therefore especially suitable for patients with sexual symptoms related to treatment. Venlafaxine is more likely to cause sexual problems than the other three drugs because it has similar properties to SSRIs at low doses. Only nefazodone is a potent inhibitor of cytochrome P450 isoenzymes. Venlafaxine, mirtazapine and reboxetine thus have very low rates of drug interactions and are potentially attractive options for patients with combined medical and psychiatric illness. However, although the efficacy of these drugs has been established they have not been evaluated specifically in medically ill populations. At present they should be used as second line drugs, to be used when SSRIs have not been effective. For further information, please see the British National Formulary (www.bnf.vhn.net).

Assessment of outcome

Once antidepressants have been prescribed it is important for the clinician to monitor the patient to assess response to treatment and potential side effects. The initial diagnosis of depression should have been made on the basis of a clinical interview, but in the context of a busy medical clinic it may be helpful for progress to be monitored by self-report questionnaire which the patient can complete while waiting to be seen. A number of well-validated instruments exist including:

▶ General Health Questionnaire[6]

▶ Hospital Anxiety and Depression Scale[7]

▶ Beck Depression Inventory[8]

▶ The Geriatric Depression Scale.[9]

Serial administration of the questionnaire gives a useful indication of response to treatment. It is recommended that clinicians familiarise themselves with the questionnaire which best suits their patients. The questionnaires are not suitable for patients with severe communication problems, for example following stroke.

5.7   More specialised psychological interventions

Patients who have been assessed as having serious psychological problems should be referred for more specialised intervention by an appropriately trained psychologist or psychiatrist. They may be able to offer a range of interventions as shown in Box 5.2.

Box 5.2   Skilled interventions which may be offered by a trained psychologist/psychiatrist

▶ Deep relaxation/autohypnosis (for generalised anxiety/tension)
▶ Systematic desensitisation and biofeedback (for specific phobias)
▶ Dynamic psychotherapy
▶ Cognitive behaviour therapy

The psychological treatments most commonly available in the NHS are cognitive behaviour therapy (CBT), counselling, psychodynamic psychotherapy, family therapy and group therapy.

Cognitive behaviour therapy is a brief, problem-oriented approach that includes behaviour therapy and cognitive therapy in various combinations. Behaviour therapy seeks to change patients' feelings and behaviour by changing their negative associations with aspects of their environment or social world that are causing them difficulty. This approach has been especially effective in treating phobias, such as those associated with needles or other aspects of medical procedures. Cognitive therapy seeks to elicit and directly change the negative thoughts and beliefs that mediate distress and problematic behaviours.

Cognitive behaviour therapy has been shown to reduce the severity of anxiety, depression, anger, obsessions, pain and a range of behavioural problems, for example eating and sleeping problems and non-adherence to advice about health. It forms an important part of self-management programmes for patients with chronic illnesses, including diabetes, arthritis and asthma. Patients are encouraged to examine the impact of their illness on their life and the way they behave, and to develop practical coping strategies to modify their behaviour, thus minimising the effects of the illness. Reported benefits of this approach include reduction of disability, improved social activity and perception of health, and reduced use of health services.[10] Most CBT is conducted by clinical psychologists or nurses who have undergone appropriate training.

Counselling is mainly available through primary care, although some departments in general hospitals, for example oncology and HIV medicine, have established their own counselling services. It is indicated for those who are having difficulty adjusting to their illness and those with relationship or interpersonal problems. It is also helpful for patients about to undergo a complicated medical procedure or an investigation which may have profound implications if the result is positive.

Psychodynamic psychotherapy aims to resolve the unconscious conflicts that are thought to underlie symptoms. It is usually a long-term treatment, sometimes taking several years, and is not available in all NHS services.

In an ideal world, psychological approaches should be used in conjunction with drug treatment but, at present, psychology services are thinly spread within the NHS. Many physicians are unaware of these facilities or do not have access to them for their patients. Valuable sources of information regarding local services include:

▸ the liaison psychiatry service

▸ the local mental health team – including community psychiatric nurses (CPNs)

▸ self-help groups

▸ local primary care trusts (PCTs).

5.8   When to refer to a psychiatrist or psychologist

Most patients with psychological problems are managed successfully by a multidisciplinary medical team. For a minority of patients with more serious problems, it is necessary to seek expert help from a mental health team. Boxes 5.3

and 5.4 list the circumstances under which it is appropriate to refer on to these professionals.

Box 5.3   Referral to a psychiatrist

Referral to a psychiatrist is necessary when:

▶ the clinician is faced with a difficult diagnostic problem (eg whether a treatable psychiatric disorder is present in a patient with unexplained physical symptoms)

▶ it is unclear whether an antidepressant might benefit a patient and, if so, which drug to choose

▶ psychiatric illness has not responded to treatment (eg antidepressants, or anxiety management)

▶ the patient poses a significant risk of deliberate self-harm

▶ there is an overt behavioural management problem (eg psychosis)

▶ further management requires follow-up and continued care from the community-based psychiatric team

▶ there is doubt about the patient's mental capacity for consent or the need for treatment under the Mental Health Act 1983

▶ there is persistent misuse of drugs or alcohol

Box 5.4   Referral to a psychologist

Referral to a psychologist is necessary when:

▶ the patient's emotional response to illness is disproportionate

▶ there is non-adherence to treatment or health advice

▶ there is a phobic response to illness or treatment

▶ the patient has difficulty coping with the demands of illness or treatment

▶ there are negative beliefs regarding illness or treatment

The suggestion of referral to a psychiatrist or psychologist may offend some patients and be resisted or flatly rejected. However, if the physician has performed a psychological assessment and possibly commenced psychiatric treatment, the suggestion that a colleague is being called in because of his/her greater expertise is logical and easy to explain. Some patients have to be specifically reassured that psychiatric referral does not indicate that they are 'mad' or 'hopeless', or that their symptoms are imaginary. The more readily available the psychiatrist and the more closely the physician and psychiatrist work together, the easier the referral.

5.9   Complementary techniques and treatment

Patients and their families frequently ask about the use of complementary measures including yoga, acupuncture, massage and aromatherapy. These should not be regarded as primary treatments. While there is little firm evidence that these have any effect on the underlying disease process, they may offer the following benefits:

> ▶ relief of tension and anxiety
> ▶ the sense of a positive action taken by the patient
> ▶ consequent improvement in well-being and quality of life.

Where these are provided privately, it is important that patients and their families are informed realistically of their likely benefits, and are not misled into the expectation of a 'miraculous cure' by unscrupulous practitioners. However, administered through registered practitioners working responsibly in partnership with traditional healthcare services, complementary therapies can form a valuable contribution to the care of chronically ill patients.

5.10   Managing sexual problems in patients with medical illness

Relationship and sexual counselling

Patients adapting to a new illness have to come to terms with many adverse social changes. Many also face a change in their marital/partnership role, particularly when the previously dominant individual is now dependent on a partner for care. For both patient and partner, this may have an impact on their sex life. Re-establishing a sexual relationship following illness is often an important goal for the patient, but is often ignored by the medical staff.

There are a number of barriers to providing sexual counselling as a routine part of medical management. These include:

> ▶ reticence – on the part of both patient and staff
> ▶ lack of time and appropriate training for staff
> ▶ lack of awareness of resources available
> ▶ lack of funding
> ▶ presumptions that older people do not have a sex life.

Initial sexual counselling often falls to the doctor who has little or no training in this area of medicine. It is helpful for the doctor to be able at least to open discussion of the subject, thereby giving the patient and partner permission to explore further if they wish, and then to know where to refer for further help and support. An approach for this is outlined below (see also Chapter 3, Section 3.10).

Is it safe to resume sexual relations?

Patients will often start by asking whether it is safe to resume sex. The advice given should take account of the following:

▶ The effects of exercise and rising blood pressure during sexual activity. Also, many drugs and diseases can cause erectile dysfunction.

▶ The importance of establishing appropriate precautions for contraception and safe sex. However, oral contraceptives may interact with certain medications, eg anticonvulsants. Also, barrier methods such as condoms or a diaphragm require dexterity, memory and motivation to apply.

Once it is established that the benefits of resuming sexual activity outweigh the risks, the patient needs to be reassured to this effect. However, the medical condition may require a change in sexual practice, and the couple may need encouragement to explore alternatives. They should be encouraged to talk to one another, to experiment with different techniques and to try other methods if one fails.

How to talk about it and with whom

Ideally, counselling should be undertaken with the patient and partner as a couple, but it is often best to see each individually at first. At the outset it is important to make sure that you have the right people – it may not be their spouse with whom they wish to resume sex.

Background information required

Patients are often unable to extrapolate information. In order to give them the particular advice they need, it is necessary to have a clear picture of their situation. It is helpful to know the answers to the following questions:

▶ What is the patient's sexual orientation? Conventional sex education often ignores homosexuality.

▶ Was the patient sexually active before?
   – if not, what was the reason?
   – do both partners acknowledge the problems?
   – do they both want a sexual relationship?

▶ Concerning their previous practice and preferences, what was important to them?

General advice

In an intimate personal relationship there are many ways of giving and receiving pleasure. It is often best to start with advice about non-penetrative sex which may be less daunting and less likely to fail.

Different positions may be recommended when the usual preferred position is impossible, or difficult to sustain for long enough to reach orgasm. This subject can be especially difficult for older couples who may see different positions as abnormal. They need to be reassured that no position is abnormal if it is mutually acceptable and that many couples use a variety of positions.

5.11   Drug treatments for erectile dysfunction

Where erectile dysfunction is the problem, specific drug treatment may be helpful both for diagnosis and management. Erectile dysfunction may have vascular, neurological, endocrine or psychological causes. Even where it has a clear pathological basis, psychological reaction (loss of confidence due to fear of failure) may exacerbate the problem. If there is no response to brief psychological intervention then physical treatments may be considered. All drug therapy should be used with caution in patients with anatomical deformity of the penis (eg Peyronie's disease) and with known cardiovascular or cerebrovascular pathology.

Oral and sublingual agents

Oral treatment with sildenafil is becoming the first line of treatment. Sildenafil produces relaxation of smooth muscle in the cavernous vessel walls, enhancing blood flow to the penis. It requires intact reflex pathways and the presence of physical and psychological sexual stimulation. It can be prescribed on the NHS only for men with certain conditions, but can be prescribed privately in other circumstances. Generalised vasodilation can lead to cardiovascular side effects, and it is contraindicated following recent stroke or myocardial infarction, or with concurrent prescription of nitrates. Headache, flushing, nasal congestion and dizziness are common side effects, but priapism is relatively rare. Patients should be warned that serious problems, including heart attack, stroke and sudden death, have been reported in temporal association with use of sildenafil. However, there is still debate about whether these are due to the drug itself or the unaccustomed sexual excitation and activity. There appears to be a 'learning curve', and the current recommendation is for patients to try up to eight times before concluding whether or not sildenifil is effective.

Sildenafil has a slow onset of action (approximately one hour) which can reduce spontaneity. Apomorphine has a faster onset of action (approximately

20 minutes) and is given sublingually. It has a similar side-effect profile. Alternative approaches may be used especially where reflex pathways are damaged, and a direct effect is required. These include alprostadil given by intracavernosal injection, or Muse® given by urethral application. Priapism is a recognised risk. Patients are best referred to a specialist sexual dysfunction clinic if these drugs are being considered.

Reporting back

Encouraging patient and partner to report back after their first two or three attempts provides reassurance that further support is on hand. At this point it is important to establish the nature of any failure. This will provide information for referral to specialist services (see Sources of further sexual counselling below).

References

1 Johnston M, Vogele C. Benefits of psychological preparation for surgery. *Ann Behav Med* 1993;**15**:245–56.

2 Gill D, Hatcher S. Antidepressants for depression in medical illness (*Cochrane Review*). *The Cochrane Library* 2002;**4**. Oxford: Update Software.

3 Anderson IM, Edwards JG. Guidelines for choice of selective serotonin reuptake inhibitor in depressive illness. *Adv Psychiat Treatment* 2001;**7**:170–80.

4 Anderson IM, Nutt DJ, Deakin JFW. Evidence-based guidelines for treating depressive disorders with antidepressants: a revision of the 1993 British Association for Psychopharmacology guidelines. *J Psychopharmacol* 2001;**14**:3–20.

5 Kent JM. SNaRIs, NaSSAs, and NaRIs: new agents for the treatment of depression. *Lancet* 2000;**355**:911–18.

6 Goldberg DP. *The detection of psychiatric illness by questionnaire.* Oxford: Oxford University Press, 1972.

7 Zigmond A, Snaith R. The hospital anxiety and depression scale. *Acta Psychiat Scand* 1983;**67**:361–70.

8 Beck AT, Ward CH, Mendelssohn MJ, Erbaugh J. An inventory for measuring depression. *Arch Gen Psychiat* 1961;**4**:561–71.

9 Brink TL, Yesavage JA, Lum O, Heersema PH, Adey M. Screening tests for geriatric depression. *Clin Gerontol* 1982;**1**:37–43.

10 Lorig KR, Sobel DS, Stewart AL. Evidence suggesting that a chronic disease self-management programme can improve health status while reducing hospitalisation. *Med Care* 1999; **37**:5–14.

Further reading

White CA. *Cognitive behaviour therapy for chronic medical problems: a guide to assessment and treatment in practice.* Chichester: Wiley, 2001.

Sources of further sexual/relationship counselling

SPOD (Association to Aid the Sexual and Personal Relationships of People with a
Disability)
Telephone sexual counselling for people with disabilities.
Tel: 020 7607 8851
Website: www.spod-uk.org

Relate
Telephone or face-to-face sexual and relationship counselling.
Tel: 01788 573241
Website: www.relate.org.uk

British Association for Sexual and Relationship Therapy
Can provide advice on registered private and other therapists.
Tel: 020 8543 2707
Website: www.basrt.org.uk

6 Deliberate self-harm

SUMMARY

▶ Deliberate self-harm (DSH) is a very common reason for hospital presentation, with approximately 140,000 cases per year in England and Wales.

▶ Many DSH patients have psychiatric and/or personality disorders. Depression and substance abuse are also common. Many patients are facing problems in relationships, socio-economic and practical difficulties, or social isolation.

▶ Episodes of deliberate self-harm are often repeated and are important precursors of suicide.

▶ Adequate clinical assessment should be conducted in all cases, either by specialist psychiatric staff or by general hospital staff. Aftercare will often involve several agencies and require careful coordination.

▶ Multidisciplinary DSH services should be developed in all large general hospitals and a DSH planning group established.

6.1 The nature of deliberate self-harm and suicide

There is controversy concerning the terminology used for non-fatal acts of deliberate self-poisoning or self-injury. 'Deliberate self-harm' (DSH)[1] will be used here. DSH has been an increasing problem in the UK, with an estimated 140,000 cases presenting to general hospitals in England and Wales each year[2] (Box 6.1). The majority of episodes involve self-poisoning, commonly with analgesics or psychotropic agents. Suicidal intent (the extent to which a person wished to die) can vary greatly and may not be reflected in the physical danger of the act. Many people are unaware of the relative dangers of different types of medication taken in overdose, so physical danger should not be assumed to indicate intent. The other frequent method of DSH is self-cutting, usually with little threat to life. A minority of episodes, however, involve deep cutting which endangers major blood vessels or nerves.

> **Box 6.1   The nature of deliberate self-harm**
>
> ▶ DSH is more common in females than males (although the gender ratio has narrowed).
>
> ▶ Rates are highest in young people, especially teenage females and young adult males. Two-thirds of patients are under 35 years of age.
>
> ▶ Rates are higher in lower socio-economic groups, the unemployed and the permanently sick.
>
> ▶ Repetition of DSH is common. At least half of DSH patients have a history of a prior episode; 15–25% will repeat DSH within a year. Some individuals carry out a large number of DSH acts.
>
> ▶ The risk of suicide is approximately 1% in the year after a DSH episode (100 times the general population risk). 40–60% of suicides have a history of DSH, with 20–25% having an episode in the year before death.

Suicide is far less common than DSH, with approximately 5,000 cases (including open verdicts) per year in England and Wales. Suicide is more common in males than females, but rates are now similar in different age groups. Many of the factors associated with suicidal behaviour are common to both DSH and suicide (see Box 6.2). However, physical illness or disability and bereavement are more commonly associated with suicide.

6.2   National suicide prevention target and strategy

There is a national target for suicide reduction for England:[3]

> Reduction in level of suicide (suicides and open verdicts) by 20% by the year 2010 (from 1995–1997 baseline)

In addition, a national suicide prevention strategy has been developed.[4] A key element in the prevention of suicide is improved management of DSH patients presenting to general hospitals. In addition to the significant risk of suicide following DSH, other reasons for this strategy include the wide variation between hospitals in the clinical approaches adopted (eg in the proportions of DSH patients admitted to inpatient beds; the availability of specialised DSH services), plus the significant morbidity represented by DSH. All large general hospitals should have a specific DSH service.

6.3   Need for psychosocial assessment of DSH patients

Psychosocial assessment of DSH patients is required to:

▶ detect those at risk of suicide or repetition of DSH

Box 6.2   Factors which contribute to DSH and suicide

▶ Psychiatric disorders – especially depression and substance misuse

▶ Alcohol and drug misuse

▶ Personality disorder – especially borderline and antisocial types

▶ Comorbidity of psychiatric and personality disorders

▶ Relationship problems – partners, parents, other family members

▶ Employment problems – particularly unemployment and economic instability

▶ Financial difficulties

▶ Socio-economic disadvantage – increased risk of suicidal behaviour in areas of socio-economic deprivation. DSH is strongly associated with lower socio-economic groups

▶ Social fragmentation (isolation)

▶ Loss of parents through separation or death

▶ Physical and sexual abuse

▶ Physical disorders – including chronic painful conditions, epilepsy

▶ Bereavement and loss

▶ Family history of suicidal behaviour

▶ Exposure to suicidal behaviour in friends and through the media

▶ identify patients with significant mental health problems requiring treatment

▶ decide what aftercare may be required – treatment in hospital as well as in the community.

In addition, the assessment procedure itself may have therapeutic benefits.

In spite of well-established standards,[5] the management of DSH patients in general hospitals varies widely,[6] with greater proportions receiving adequate psychosocial assessment in some hospitals than in others. Patients who are managed entirely in the accident and emergency (A&E) department without admission to a general hospital bed are particularly likely not to be assessed.[6] The National Institute for Clinical Excellence is currently developing guidelines on the management of DSH patients.

6.4   Assessment by general medical staff

All medical and nursing staff who have responsibility for the care of DSH patients should be able to carry out a rapid assessment and appraisal of risk. This is because:

▶ Patients may refuse to see a mental health specialist or leave abruptly, before a full assessment can be undertaken.

▶ Patients who leave A&E departments before they are assessed by a mental health professional have a greater likelihood of repetition of DSH than those who are assessed.[7]

▶ Even if patients are admitted for observation to a medical ward, they may decide to leave before a mental health professional can assess them.

▶ Emotional status can fluctuate dramatically following self-harm, and the risk of further self-harm can change.

The objectives of this assessment are to detect immediate suicide risk, identify severe mental illness, and determine whether patients who are refusing treatment or trying to leave the hospital are mentally fit to decline help (see Chapter 9). It is essential that when a patient leaves the hospital without a full psychosocial assessment this is rapidly communicated to their GP.

Key aspects of the assessment of suicide risk are indicated in Box 6.3. If there is any evidence from this assessment that the patient wanted to die or that suicidal plans are still prominent, it is important to try to persuade the patient to stay for a full psychosocial assessment. If this is refused, it may be necessary to detain the patient under mental health legislation for a fuller assessment. The medical team

---

Box 6.3 Assessment of immediate suicide risk

It is advisable to see the patient in a private setting and allow sufficient time to make a careful assessment. Try to start the interview by asking general questions about how the patient is feeling, in particular whether they feel low. In the context of enquiring about mood, it is natural to move to a discussion of suicidal ideation, eg *'Given that you've been feeling down, and you took an overdose of tablets, I was wondering...'*

Key areas of enquiry include:

▶ The seriousness of intent involved in the self-harm episode:
What was going through your mind when you took the tablets?
Did you intend to kill yourself?

▶ The patient's view of the survival, if there was suicidal intent:
How do you feel now that you're in hospital, and that you didn't die?
I was wondering if you have any regrets ... or whether you feel relieved?

▶ The patient's current suicidal status:
Do you still have any thoughts of harming yourself?
How strong are those thoughts?
How likely are you to act upon them?

will need to contact the psychiatric team urgently to obtain further advice. If a patient wishes to leave before a Mental Health Act assessment can be made, restraint can be applied (physically if necessary) under common law.

The assessment of capacity to refuse treatment is discussed in detail in Chapter 9. In relation to DSH, it becomes an important issue if a patient refuses medical treatment for the physical sequelae of the self-harm, which may then have potentially lethal consequences. Individuals are entitled to refuse medical treatment if they have the capacity to do so. All registered doctors should be able to assess capacity, but in cases of DSH this can be particularly difficult as capacity may be temporarily impaired by the patient's mental state. Advice should be sought from the psychiatric team. Common case scenarios in this regard are described in Chapter 9.

If the patient wants to leave before a detailed psychosocial assessment can be carried out, it is also important to enquire about the home circumstances and the degree of support available.

Figure 6.1 shows an algorithm to help medical and general nursing staff assess the risk involved when a patient wishes to leave before they have received a psycho-social assessment, and the actions that should be considered. It is meant as a general guide to aid decision-making and should not be rigidly applied in all circumstances, as individual situations will vary.

Medical or general nursing staff can be trained to conduct full psychosocial assessments, but in reality there is seldom the time available for them to do so, or the training and support available to enhance their skills. The key components of a full psychosocial assessment are described below.

6.5   Essential components of assessment procedure

Psychosocial assessment should be conducted after the patient has fully recovered from any toxic effects of DSH. Staff conducting the assessments should be adequately trained in the procedure. They should also have access to senior psychiatric advice and supervision. The assessment should be conducted in a private setting where other patients cannot overhear what is being said. Gathering of information should include interviewing relatives or other informants plus inquiry of the GP and any other clinicians already involved in care.

Topics that should be covered during the assessment are shown in Box 6.4. A structured form may aid the assessment procedure. It is important to be aware that a patient's level of distress or intent can change quickly due, for example, to the responses of relatives or friends, or other interventions. DSH in the context of a severe physical illness may sometimes appear to be an 'understandable'

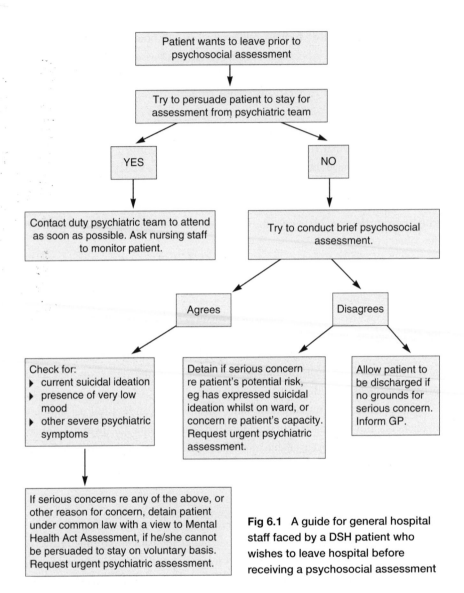

Fig 6.1 A guide for general hospital staff faced by a DSH patient who wishes to leave hospital before receiving a psychosocial assessment

reaction to the condition and its implications. However, depression (which may be treatable) is very often present.

6.6   Aftercare on discharge from the general hospital

Psychiatric hospital inpatient care is required for between 5 and 10% of DSH patients. Indications include severe psychiatric disorder and continuing risk of suicide. The majority of patients can best be helped by brief psychological treat-

> **Box 6.4 Topics that should be covered in the assessment of patients who have self-harmed**
>
> ▶ Events and problems that preceded DSH
> ▶ Suicidal intent and other motives involved in the act
> ▶ Current problems facing the patient
> ▶ Alcohol and drug use
> ▶ Current psychiatric disorder
> ▶ Personality traits and disorder
> ▶ Family and personal history
> ▶ Psychiatric history, including previous DSH (and its consequences)
> ▶ Risk of suicide
> ▶ Coping resources and available supports
> ▶ Most appropriate aftercare, and patient's willingness to accept help

ment – problem-solving therapy or a similar approach being most appropriate. Evidence is now emerging for the effectiveness of such therapy with regard to reducing risk of repetition of DSH, improving depression and hopelessness, and bringing about changes in patients' problems.[8–10] Such treatment can be provided by members of a hospital-based DSH team or of a community mental health team. Continuity of care is associated with better adherence to treatment. Psychotropic medication may also be indicated, although care must be taken to use drugs with low toxicity, and large prescriptions should be avoided because of the risk of overdose.

Many DSH patients have personality disorders (often in combination with psychiatric disorder, especially depression and/or substance abuse). Such patients may present considerable challenges in management. It is essential that help for substance misuse is readily available in the general hospital; this usually involves having staff from the local substance misuse service working closely with the medical and psychiatric teams involved in the management of DSH. Treatment of personality disorders can be extremely difficult and there is only limited evidence of efficacy of specific therapies. Good communication between all agencies involved is essential. DSH patients with combined personality and psychiatric disorders, including substance misuse, are at particularly high risk of eventual suicide. Social services have a major role in management where young children are involved, especially if risk of parental abuse or neglect is apparent. Social workers also have a significant potential role where the patient's problems include housing and accommodation difficulties, and need for benefits.

6.7   Patients who present specific management issues

Adolescents aged 16 years and over

Adolescents will often require clinical input from child and adolescent psychiatric services. There must therefore be close liaison with the local service. Many patients in this category should be admitted to a general hospital bed to allow adequate assessment, including interviews with families and possible involvement of community statutory services (eg social services). Family problem-solving therapy is often an acceptable form of treatment, although evidence regarding efficacy is still lacking. Group treatment for those who repeatedly self-harm is a promising approach for adolescents. Individual psychological therapy, found to be effective for treatment of depression in adolescents, requires investigation in young DSH patients. Where depression is marked, treatment with an antidepressant (preferably an SSRI) is indicated (see Chapter 5).

Older people

Full psychosocial assessment is recommended for all older DSH patients. DSH is less common in older people but more often associated with significant suicidal intent. The risk of subsequent suicide is particularly high in older DSH patients. Close liaison with the local old age psychiatry service is important for assessment and aftercare.

Frequent repeaters of DSH

Approximately 10–15% of DSH patients will have a history of five or more episodes of self-harm, with a small proportion having engaged in very many episodes. The motivation behind the behaviour can be difficult to discern, but the risk of eventual suicide is high in those who repeatedly self-harm. Management is also problematic as these patients often have personality disorders, typically in the antisocial, border-line or dependent categories. Comorbidity with substance misuse and affective disorder is common. Management may therefore need to include multiple agencies and requires clear communication between the clinicians involved. There is prelim-inary evidence that intensive psychological treatment ('dialectical behaviour therapy') may be helpful for patients with borderline personality disorder. Low dose neuroleptics may help reduce frequent repetition of DSH (possibly by lower-ing arousal in response to stress). In one trial, an SSRI antidepressant (paroxetine) was associated with reduced repetition of DSH in those with a history of 2–5 episodes, but because this finding was based on *post hoc* subgroup analysis it must be treated with caution.[11]

6.8 Attitudes towards DSH patients and factors that may impair adequate care

Attitudes of medical and nursing staff to DSH patients can be quite negative.[12] This may be partly because their behaviour is viewed as self-inflicted and hence they are seen as less deserving than other patients, and partly because of the clinical management problems they often pose. Repetitive DSH patients may be viewed particularly negatively. While these attitudes may in some ways be understandable, it is important that the seriousness of DSH patients' problems and suicidal behaviour be acknowledged and understood. This is a group with a risk of suicide very many times higher than that of the general population. Their behaviour represents considerable psychosocial morbidity and distress. Often their problems result from socio-economic disadvantage and damaging experiences during their upbringing. Genetics and family history are also important contributory factors.

DSH patients are often aware of negative attitudes of staff, and their consequent hostility towards staff can make management all the more difficult. Empathic efforts to understand the patients' difficulties in the context of their life experience may improve management. Admitting most DSH patients who require hospital admission to a short-stay ward can also be helpful. This means that the ward staff get considerable experience of these patients, and liaison and communication with psychiatric staff are usually enhanced.

6.9 DSH services

Increasing numbers of general hospitals are developing special psychiatric services for DSH patients, often as part of an overall liaison psychiatry service. These usually incorporate psychiatrically trained nurses, social workers, and, sometimes, clinical psychologists working with psychiatrists. There is good evidence that adequately trained nonmedical staff are able to conduct psychosocial assessments of equivalent quality to those of psychiatrists.[13] Liaison psychiatry nurses have assumed a leading role in this respect. The introduction of a DSH service results in shortened length of inpatient admissions.[14] Many services have to rely on the local on-call psychiatric service at night and often at weekends. The desirable staffing level of a DSH service is indicated in Chapter 10.

In the Royal College of Psychiatrists' guidelines, *The general hospital management of adult deliberate self-harm,*[5] the response times recommended for assessment by specialist staff are as shown in Box 6.5.

It is advisable that a DSH service planning group is established to enhance the care of DSH patients and to ensure good communication between the relevant

---

Box 6.5 Recommended response times for assessment by DSH service staff[4]

Inpatients

Non-urgent cases should be seen for assessment:

▸ on the same working day if the referral is made from the ward during the first part of the morning

▸ within 24 hours if the request comes later in the day

Patients in A&E

▸ DSH patients should not be required to wait in A&E for more than 3 hours

▸ A&E staff should have immediate access to telephone advice from a member of a self-harm specialist team or from a psychiatrist whose duties include advice to, and attendance at, A&E

▸ A request for emergency attendance at A&E should result in the arrival of a member of the self-harm specialist team or a duty psychiatrist within an hour

---

clinical services involved in care and with hospital managers. This group can assess local needs, identify the necessary level of staffing of the service, review its functioning, attend to links and relationships with other services, develop policy documents, investigate problems that may arise and plan future projects and developments. The potential representatives of such a group are shown in Box 6.6.

6.10 Audit and research

DSH services are strongly encouraged to audit their work. In addition to monitoring number of patients and workload, the service might, for example, review the

---

Box 6.6 Potential members of a DSH service planning group

▸ Representatives (medical and nonmedical) of the DSH service

▸ Representatives (medical and nursing) of the A&E department

▸ Representatives of general medical ward staff

▸ Member of child and adolescent psychiatric service

▸ Member of old age psychiatry service

▸ Member of alcohol and drugs service

▸ Hospital manager

▸ Primary care representative

▸ Representatives of local Samaritans and other crisis agencies

▸ Representative of an appropriate users' group

proportions of DSH patients who present to the hospital and receive a psychosocial assessment, investigate views of patients on the care received, the satisfaction of A&E and general medical staff with the service, and identify aspects of care or specific groups of patients which require further attention.

There is a considerable need for more research on DSH, particularly evaluation of different types of management and aftercare. Such studies often require relatively large numbers of patients in order to provide substantive findings, so research collaboration between DSH services in different hospitals is desirable.

References

1 NHS Centre For Reviews and Dissemination. Effective Health Care Bulletin: Deliberate self-harm. *Effective Health Care* 1998;4:1–12.

2 Hawton K, Arensman E, Townsend E, Bremner S *et al.* Deliberate self-harm: systematic review of efficacy of psychosocial and pharmacological treatments in preventing repetition. *BMJ* 1998;317:441–7.

3 Department of Health (1999). *Saving lives: our healthier nation: a contract for health*, Cm 4386. London: The Stationery Office.

4 Department of Health. *National suicide prevention strategy for England*. London: DH, 2002. www.doh.gov.uk/mentalhealth/suicideprevention.htm

5 Royal College of Psychiatrists. *The general hospital management of adult deliberate self-harm*. Council Report CR32. London: Royal College of Psychiatrists, 1994.

6 Kapur N, House A., Creed F, Feldman E *et al.* Management of deliberate self poisoning in adults in four teaching hospitals: descriptive study. *BMJ* 1998;316:831–2.

7 Hickey L, Hawton K, Fagg J, Weitzel H. Deliberate self-harm patients who leave the accident and emergency department without a psychiatric assessment. A neglected population at risk of suicide. *J Psychosom Res* 2001;50:87–93.

8 Hawton K, Fagg J, Simkin, S, Bale E, Bond A. Trends in deliberate self-harm in Oxford, 1985-1995. Implications for clinical services and the prevention of suicide. *Br J Psychiat* 1997;171:556–60.

9 Guthrie E, Kapur N, Mackway-Jones K, Chew-Graham C *et al.* Randomised controlled trial of brief psychological intervention after deliberate self poisoning. *BMJ* 2001;323:135–7.

10 Townsend E, Hawton K, Altman DG, Arensman E *et al.* The efficacy of problem-solving treatments after deliberate self-harm: meta-analysis of randomized controlled trials with respect to depression, hopelessness and improvement in problems. *Psychol Med* 2001;31:979–88.

11 Verkes R, Cowen P. Pharmacotherapy of suicidal ideation and behaviour. In Hawton K, van Heeringen K (eds), *The international handbook of suicide and attempted suicide*. Chichester: Wiley, 2000: 487–502.

12 Hemmings A. Attitudes to deliberate self harm among staff in an accident and emergency team. *Mental Health Care* 1999;2:300–302.

13 Catalan J, Marsack P, Hawton K, Whitwell, D *et al.* Comparison of doctors and nurses in the assessment of deliberate self-poisoning patients. *Psychol Med* 1980; 10:483–91.

14 Hawton K, Gath DH, Smith EBO. Management of attempted suicide in Oxford. *BMJ* 1979;ii:1040–42.

Further reading

NHS Centre for Reviews and Dissemination. Effective Health Care Bulletin: Deliberate self-harm. *Effective Health Care* 1998;**4**:1–12.

Hawton K. General hospital management of suicide attempters. In Hawton K, Van Heeringen K (eds) *The international handbook of suicide and attempted suicide.* Chichester: Wiley, 2000:519–37.

Hawton K, Catalan J. *Attempted suicide: a practical guide to its nature and management,* 2nd edn. Oxford: Oxford University Press, 1987.

7 | Alcohol and drug misuse

SUMMARY

▶ Alcohol and drug misuse are common in general hospital patients. Screening tests are easy to use and improve detection.

▶ Basic alcohol and drug detoxification is straightforward; complex cases should be supported by specialist advice. Thiamine should be given parenterally in alcohol detoxification.

▶ Structured, brief interventions can be delivered by any member of the general hospital team after appropriate training.

▶ Specialist substance misuse liaison teams can offer support and training as well as direct intervention.

▶ More undergraduate and postgraduate training in substance misuse issues should be provided.

7.1 Introduction

Alcohol misuse contributes to 20–25% of all general hospital admissions.[1,2] The question 'Alcohol – can the NHS afford it?' is answered by the key recommendation that 'the widespread consequences of alcohol misuse in this country should be given a higher profile', including a 'defined hospital strategy'.[3] Alcohol misuse is a risk factor for many serious conditions, including cancers, heart disease and stroke, accidents, and suicide, which are the four national targets in *Saving lives: our healthier nation*.[4] Despite the incontrovertible evidence in support of a national alcohol strategy, none has yet been produced.[5]

Drug misuse is being addressed through *Tackling drugs to build a better Britain*,[6] which outlines the Government's ten-year strategy and has four key target domains:

▶ to help young people resist drug use

▶ to protect communities from drug-related antisocial and criminal behaviour

▶ to enable people with drug problems to overcome them and live healthy and crime-free lives

▶ to stem the availability of illegal drugs.

It is being implemented through a new special health authority, the National Treatment Agency, with responsibility for pooled treatment funds for drug misuse. It does not have responsibility yet for alcohol and has focused mainly on prevention and community safety issues, with negligible attention to the burden placed on secondary healthcare.

Smoking causes one in every five deaths in the UK and the loss of more than 550,000 years before the age of 75,[7] but is not within the remit of this document.

7.2   Definitions

A unit of alcohol is 8g of ethanol which is contained in:

▶ a half pint of normal strength beer, lager or cider

▶ a quarter pint of extra strong beer, lager or cider

▶ a small (125 ml) glass of wine

▶ a 50 ml glass of sherry or port

▶ a single pub measure (25 ml) of spirits.

Sensible drinking is up to 21 units for men or 14 units for women, weekly, spread over four or more days. Drinking above these levels is termed 'alcohol misuse'. Hazardous drinking occurs at above 35 units per week for men and 21 units for women. Dependence is more likely above 50 units per week for men and 35 units for women. The term 'alcoholic' should be avoided as it is poorly defined and pejorative.

Drug misuse describes any unsanctioned use of a psychoactive substance. Dependence has physical and psychological components. Some classes of drug do not have marked features of physical dependence (physical withdrawal symptoms or tolerance).

7.3   Screening

It is easy to screen general hospital patients for drug and alcohol misuse. It is important to avoid stereotyping patients because people of all age groups and walks of life may exhibit these problems. The presenting problem and physical examination may indicate that there is a high likelihood of substance misuse, but, for most patients, structured questioning may help to overcome any embarrassment. The one-minute Paddington Alcohol Test[8] can be used in A&E to detect harmful and hazardous drinking (see Appendix 1, p.87). The Alcohol Use Disorders Identification Test (AUDIT)[9] may be used alone or as part of enquiry about lifestyle, and covers amount and frequency of drinking, indicators of alcohol dependence and common problems caused by alcohol (see Appendix 2, p.88).

The CAGE questionnaire[10] is short and simple but relatively insensitive to milder, hazardous drinking (see Box 7.1). A positive answer to two or more questions points to an alcohol problem.

Box 7.1 The CAGE questionnaire

C Have you ever thought you ought to **C**ut down on your drinking?

A Have people **A**nnoyed you by criticising your drinking?

G Have you ever felt bad or **G**uilty about your drinking?

E Have you ever had a drink first thing in the morning to steady your nerves or to get rid of a hangover (an **E**ye-opener)?

The features of drug misuse depend on the classes of drug in question and whether the patient is intoxicated, in withdrawal (if there is a withdrawal syndrome), or in a more neutral state at the time of assessment. Urine drug-testing is a useful adjunct to clinical assessment. Commercially available 'dip stick' tests are available but laboratory tests (gas chromatography linked with mass spectrometry (GC-MS)) may be easier for the non-specialist to perform and interpret, provide clinical biochemistry backup, and generate a record for the case notes. Laboratory testing is limited by the availability and speed of obtaining results. The approximate durations of detectability for some of the more common drugs in circulation are shown in Appendix 3, p.90. Increasingly, patients may exhibit polydrug misuse with features of intoxication or withdrawal from more than one class of drug and from alcohol. It is important to ascertain the possibility of epileptic fits and of Wernicke-Korsakoff syndrome and to treat these prophylactically. Once drug or alcohol problems are detected, it is important to act to treat the acute situation, to take advice if necessary, and refer if appropriate.

7.4 Alcohol detoxification[11]

Alcohol enhances the inhibitory effects of gamma amino-butyric acid (GABA) and reduces excitatory N-methyl-D-aspartate (NMDA). Therefore, a GABA agonist should be given, though not chlormethiazole (except when an i.v. infusion is indicated) because of its short half-life and relative neurotoxicity with alcohol.[12] Use a long-acting benzodiazepine such as chlordiazapoxide, as shown in Table 7.1.

Table 7.1 A typical reducing schedule of chlordiazapoxide for symptomatic support

Day	Morning (mg)	Midday (mg)	Afternoon (mg)	Night (mg)	Total daily dose (mg)
1	20	20	20	20	80
2	20	15	15	20	70
3	15	15	15	15	60
4	15	10	10	15	50
5	10	10	10	10	40
6	10	5	5	10	30
7	5	5	5	5	20
8	5			5	10
9				5	5
10					Discontinue

Increased doses may be needed at first in patients with severe withdrawal.
Mild withdrawal symptoms may start at a lower dose (60 mg/day).
Beta-blockers should be used only as adjunctive therapy and never as monotherapy.

B-complex vitamins should be given for the prophylaxis and treatment of Wernicke-Korsakoff syndrome.[13] Wernicke's encephalopathy is not rare (12–34% of 'alcoholic' brains show evidence of it). The triad of ophthalmoplegia, confusion and ataxia is not invariably present (only 10% of these cases have all three). Oral thiamine is too poorly absorbed to offset Wernicke-Korsakoff syndrome, so parenteral doses should be administered (Pabrinex® ampoules 1&2, 1–2 pairs for 3–5 days, i.m. for prophylaxis/early signs, i.v. for established disorder). An allergic response occurs rarely (0.1%) and is associated slightly more often with the i.v. route than the i.m. route. There is minimal evidence of any response to thiamine in established Wernicke-Korsakoff syndrome.

Adjunctive medication includes:

▶ β-blockers for hypertension
▶ carbamazepine for seizures
▶ haloperidol for hallucinations (butyrophenones are the least epileptogenic of the major tranquillisers, but are needed rarely)
▶ thiamine and magnesium for nutritional deficiency.

7.5   Drug detoxification

Drug detoxification is required when there is objective evidence of physical withdrawal and usually only applies to opioids and sedative-hypnotics. It relies on accurate detection of symptoms and signs and, if possible, on corroborative information. Mild opioid withdrawal can be treated symptomatically with anxiolytic and antidiarrhoeal medication. Otherwise, opioid substitution should be offered after consultation with a liaison and/or an addiction psychiatrist. Oral methadone mixture is offered as it is easily supervised and longer acting. Typically, 5–10 mg oral methadone is a reasonable starting dose. Although liable to being crushed and injected, dihydrocodeine tablets may be used as an interim measure, titrated against the relief of objective features of withdrawal and observing for evidence of toxicity and overdosage. Box 7.2 gives signs of opioid intoxication and Box 7.3 shows symptoms and signs of withdrawal.[14] The grading of the abstinence syndrome allows an assessment of the severity of physical dependence and the need for treatment.

Box 7.2   Signs of opioid intoxication

▶ Euphoria/relaxation

▶ Feeling of well-being

▶ Constricted pupils

▶ Drowsiness

▶ Slurred speech

▶ Poor attention and concentration

Box 7.3   Opioid abstinence syndrome: symptoms and signs

Grade 0:   Drug craving
　　　　　 Anxiety
　　　　　 Drug-seeking behaviour

Grade 1:   Yawning
　　　　　 Sweating
　　　　　 Running eyes and nose
　　　　　 Restless sleep

Grade 2:   Dilated pupils
　　　　　 Goose flesh ('cold turkey')
　　　　　 Hot and cold flushes:
　　　　　　 shivering
　　　　　 Aching bones and
　　　　　　 muscles
　　　　　 Loss of appetite
　　　　　 Irritability

Grade 3:   Insomnia
　　　　　 Low-grade fever
　　　　　 Increased pulse rate
　　　　　 Increased blood pressure
　　　　　 Increased respiratory rate
　　　　　 Restlessness
　　　　　 Abdominal cramps
　　　　　 Nausea and vomiting
　　　　　 Diarrhoea
　　　　　 Weakness
　　　　　 Weight loss

Sedative-hypnotic withdrawal is treated with long-acting benzodiazepines (Table 7.2) as for alcohol withdrawal, although the length of the detoxification may be increased after consultation. Anticonvulsants may be necessary if there is a history of epileptiform fits. Patients may become anxious and/or demanding and it is very important to treat only their objective signs, with appropriate management of their psychological distress and/or disturbance as for any other patient.

Sedative-hypnotic abstinence symptoms are shown in Box 7.4.

Where there is no marked physical withdrawal syndrome (eg for stimulants and cannabinoids), there may be psychological features that require general support. In particular, sudden cessation of stimulant medication can lead to extreme low mood with risks of deliberate self-harm that should be managed as for any suicidal patient.

Table 7.2 Approximate dose equivalents for benzodiazepines[15]

Drug	Dose equivalent (mg)
Diazepam	5
Chlordiazepoxide	25
Flurazepam	15
Lorazepam	1
Nitrazepam	2.5
Temazepam	20

Box 7.4 Sedative-hypnotic abstinence symptoms and signs

- Anxiety
- Tremor
- Poor concentration
- Insomnia
- Nausea and vomiting
- Sweating
- Paraesthesia and muscle aches

- Hypersensitivity to sensory stimuli
- Perceptual distortions
- Depersonalisation
- Depression
- Epileptiform seizures
- Delirium

7.6 Comorbid substance misuse and psychiatric disorder ('dual diagnosis')

Substance misuse and psychiatric disorder can occur together in a number of ways:[16]

- primary mental illness with subsequent (consequent) substance misuse

▶ primary substance misuse with psychiatric sequelae

▶ dual primary diagnosis

▶ common aetiological factors causing mental illness and substance misuse.

After affective disorder, substance misuse is the single most important variable in completed suicide: 40% of cases have a history of alcohol misuse and 28% have a history of drug misuse[17] although these are the primary diagnoses in only 9% and 4% of cases respectively. The nature of the interaction is complex, and pragmatic approaches must be used to minimise risks and prevent such patients 'falling through the net'. The Mental Health Act 1983 excludes substance misuse *per se* but can be used to detain patients compulsorily if, for example, depressive features are present, on the basis that an affective disorder and substance misuse may (and do commonly) coexist. However, local arrangements and protocols should be in place to deal with patients who appear to be intoxicated, in which case detailed medical and psychiatric assessment may need to be delayed.

Detailed discussion[18] is beyond the scope of this document but effective management of this large group of patients depends on collaborative approaches between teams and the use of proper care planning mechanisms.

7.7   Effective interventions for substance misusers

In the general hospital, management of intoxication, overdose and withdrawal remains the most important objective. However, brief interventions by non-specialists have a proven benefit in reducing alcohol intake by about 20% for general hospital patients.[3] There is usually an assessment of alcohol intake, information on hazardous drinking and clear advice, often supported by patient information and details of local services. The elements of effective brief interventions are encapsulated in the acronym FRAMES (Box 7.5).[19]

The evidence supporting brief interventions for drug misuse is less clear, but the principles of assessment and information-giving appear robust. In particular, clear

---

Box 7.5   FRAMES

F   Feedback on personal risk or impairment
R   Emphasis on personal **R**esponsibility for change
A   Clear **A**dvice on how to change
M   A **M**enu of alternative change options
E   Therapeutic **E**mpathy as a counselling style
S   Enhancement of patient **S**elf-efficacy or optimism

advice should be given about where to seek treatment. Community drug (and alcohol) teams provide assessment and treatment and should be one of the first-line options, along with non-statutory agencies and self-help groups. Increasingly, GPs are undergoing training in the management of drug misusers and many more are available to offer treatment than hitherto, with support from local specialist services.

Motivational interviewing[20] is a powerful cognitive behavioural technique to deal with denial and ambivalence in people with substance misuse (or any other health condition where there is resistance to accepting appropriate help). It uses a cyclical model to describe phases of motivation (see Fig 7.1),[21] helps the patient to draw up a 'balance sheet' of the pros and cons of receiving treatment, and recognises and tackles ambivalence and relapse as anticipated phenomena.

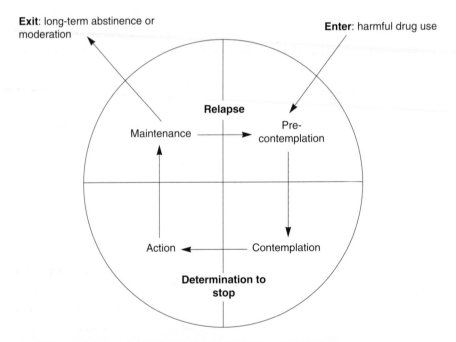

Fig 7.1 Stages of change (Prochaska and DiClemente, 1986).[21]

Relapse prevention[22] provides an effective model for promoting remission, using a range of cognitive, behavioural and social interventions:

▸ identification of high-risk relapse factors

▸ understanding relapse as both a process and as an event

▸ dealing with substance cues as well as with craving

▶ dealing with social pressures to use drugs

▶ development of supportive networks

▶ coping with negative emotional states

▶ development of plans to interrupt a lapse or relapse.

Medication has a small role in relapse prevention and can be given as an early adjunct to psychosocial treatment. In alcohol dependence syndrome, acamprosate (and, perhaps, naltrexone) may help to reduce craving for alcohol when used in this way. For fully detoxified and motivated patients with opioid dependence, naltrexone is effective in reducing the chances that a lapse (ie a few instances of opioid use without the re-establishment of dependence) will lead to a full-blown relapse.

Specialist substance misuse treatment services provide a source of advice, training, support and information as well as direct intervention (Useful contacts, p.92). There are a small number of dedicated teams working within general hospitals to complement liaison psychiatry services and to provide proactive responses to the large number of patients with clinically significant substance misuse. There is robust evidence for a range of specialist interventions being effective in reducing harm to drug misusers.[23] For alcohol, Project MATCH (the largest ever study of psychological interventions for alcohol misuse) showed that abstinence-based approaches are effective.[24] These are effective counter-arguments to the nihilism that can still hinder the detection and treatment of substance misusers.

7.8 Special issues

Communicable diseases

Substance misuse in general and injecting drug misuse use in particular carry with them significant risks of Hepatitis B, Hepatitis C and HIV.[25] This is linked to unsafe sexual practices as well as 'sharing' injecting equipment and should be included in the assessment of substance misusers' physical and psychological states.

Obstetric and neonatal complications

The spectrum of fetal alcohol effects is under-recognised. Despite sometimes chaotic use of antenatal services, the intrauterine effects of maternal cocaine misuse (leading to 'crack babies') can be offset by early detection and intervention. Neonatal opioid withdrawal as well as HIV transmission also have to be borne in mind. Child protection issues are paramount.

Young people

The specific needs of young people are addressed by the Health Advisory Service 2000 report[26] which indicates the need for substance misuse services specifically for young people, and the importance of collaborative working with, *inter alia*, paediatric and child and adolescent mental health services.

Accident and emergency departments

Accident and emergency departments provide an ideal opportunity for screening and intervention for substance misuse.[27] Also, issues of safety should be addressed to ensure that both patients and staff know that inappropriate behaviour will not be tolerated.

Education and training

Substance misuse in general hospitals is a common phenomenon, which can be screened for, and is amenable to brief as well as specialist interventions. There is therefore a clear case for greater undergraduate and postgraduate training to give medical and other hospital staff the knowledge, skills and perspective to play their part in tackling the problem.

APPENDIX 1   The one-minute Paddington Alcohol Test (PAT)[8]

After dealing with the patient's reasons for attendance at A&E, ask the following questions:

1   *Quite a number of people have times when they drink more than usual; what is the most you will drink in any one day?*
    (Note: 1 unit = 8 g alcohol. Units contained in pub measures are given in brackets; home measures of 'singles', for example, are often three times greater than a pub measure.)

Beer/lager/cider	☐ Pints (2)	☐ Cans (1.5)
Strong beer/lager/cider	☐ Pints (5)	☐ Cans (4)
Wine	☐ Glasses (1.5)	☐ Bottles (9)
Fortified wine (sherry, martini)	☐ Glasses (1)	☐ Bottles (12)
Spirits (gin, whisky, vodka)	☐ Singles (1)	☐ Bottles (30)

Total units/day = ☐

2   *If you sometimes drink more than 8 units/day* (for men), *or 6 units/day* (for women), *is this at least once a week?*

Yes = PAT +ve
No = *Go to* Question 3

3   *Do you feel your current attendance at A&E is related to alcohol?*

Yes = PAT +ve
No = PAT –ve

Patients who are PAT +ve should be offered specific alcohol advice and managed according to local protocol.

APPENDIX 2   The Alcohol Use Disorders Identification Test (AUDIT) questionnaire

Circle the number that comes closest to the patient's answer.

1 *How often do you have a drink containing alcohol?**

(0) Never	(1) Monthly or less	(2) Two to four times a month	(3) Two to three times a week	(4) Four or more times a week

2 *How many drinks containing alcohol do you have on a typical day when you are drinking?* (Code number of standard drinks.)*

(0) 1 or 2	(1) 3 or 4	(2) 5 or 6	(3) 7 or 8	(4) 10 or more

3 *How often do you have six or more drinks on one occasion?*

(0) Never	(1) Less than monthly	(2) Monthly	(3) Weekly	(4) Daily or almost daily

4 *How often during the last year have you found that you were not able to stop drinking once you had started?*

(0) Never	(1) Less than monthly	(2) Monthly	(3) Weekly	(4) Daily or almost daily

5 *How often during the last year have you failed to do what was normally expected of you because of drinking?*

(0) Never	(1) Less than monthly	(2) Monthly	(3) Weekly	(4) Daily or almost daily

6 *How often during the last year have you needed a first drink in the morning to get yourself going after a heavy drinking session?*

(0) Never	(1) Less than monthly	(2) Monthly	(3) Weekly	(4) Daily or almost daily

7 *How often during the last year have you had a feeling of guilt or remorse after drinking?*

(0) Never	(1) Less than monthly	(2) Monthly	(3) Weekly	(4) Daily or almost daily

8   *How often during the last year have you been unable to remember what*
    happened the night before because you had been drinking?

(0) Never	(1) Less than monthly	(2) Monthly	(3) Weekly	(4) Daily or almost daily

9   *Have you or someone else been injured as a result of your drinking?*

(0) No	(1) Yes, but not in the last year	(2) Yes, during the last year

10 *Has a relative of friend or a doctor or other health worker been concerned about*
    your drinking or suggested you cut down?

(0) No	(1) Yes, but not in the last year	(2) Yes, during the last year

*In determining the response categories it has been assumed that one 'drink' contains 10 g alcohol. In countries where the alcohol content of a standard drink differs by more than 25% from 10 g, the response category should be modified accordingly.

Record sum of individual item scores here: ⬜

Each item is scored 0–4, giving a maximum score of 40. A score of 8 or more indicates likely hazardous drinking.

APPENDIX 3   Laboratory investigations for drugs[28]

Dip sticks tests are less reliable than gas chromatography linked with mass spectrometry (GC-MS).

Drug	Approximate durations of detectability
Amphetamine	2–3 days
Methadone	7–9 days
MDMA (ecstasy)	30–48 hr
Cocaine	6–8 hr
Benzodiazepines	
Short-acting	24 hr
Intermediate-acting	40–80 hr
Long-acting	>7 days
Codeine/morphine	24 hr
Dihydrocodeine	24 hr
Buprenorphine	48-56 hr
Cannabinoids	
Single use	3 days
Moderate use	4 days
Heavy (daily) use	10 days
Chronic heavy use	<36 days

MDMA = methylenedioxymethamphetamine.

Many drugs have active metabolites which can also test positive.

Potential sources of urinary morphine include:

▶ use of codeine

▶ foodstuffs, including poppy seed strudel and cake

▶ analgesic preparations, eg Gee's linctus, kaolin and morphine mixture.

Methods of analysing saliva, breath (as for alcohol) and sweat for drug detection are being developed.

References

1   Jarman CMB, Kellett JM. Alcoholism in the general hospital. *BMJ* 1979;**ii**:469–72.
2   Lloyd GG, Chick J, Crombie E. Screening for problem drinkers among medical inpatients. *Drug Alcohol Dependence* 1982;**10**:355–9.
3   Royal College of Physicians. *Alcohol – can the NHS afford it?* Report of a working party. London: RCP, 2001.
4   Department of Health. *Saving lives: our healthier nation,* Cm 4386. London: Stationery Office, 1999.
5   Raistrick D, Ritson B, Hodgson R (eds). *Tackling alcohol together.* London: Free Association Books, 1999.
6   Home Office. *Tackling drugs to build a better Britain. The government's ten-year strategy for tackling drugs misuse,* Cm 3945. London: Stationery Office, 1998.
7   Royal College of Physicians' Tobacco Advisory Group. *Nicotine addiction in Britain.* London: RCP, 2000.
8   Smith SGT, Touquet R, Wright S, Gupta ND. Detection of alcohol misusing patients in accident and emergency departments: the Paddington Alcohol Test (PAT). *J Accid Emerg Med* 1996;**13**:591–9.
9   Harvey J. Detecting the problem drinker. *Medicine (Balt)* 1995;**23**:47–50.
10 Mayfield D, MacLeod G, Hall P. The CAGE questionnaire: validation of a new alcohol-screening instrument. *Am J Psychiat* 1974;**131**:1121–3.
11 Raistrick D. Management of alcohol detoxification. *Adv Psychiat Treatment* 2000;**6**:348–55.
12 McInnes G. Chlormethiazole and alcohol: a lethal cocktail. *BMJ* 1987;**294**:592.
13 Cook CC, Thompson AD. B-complex vitamins in the treatment and prophylaxis of Wernicke-Korsakoff syndrome. *Br J Hosp Med* 1997;**57**:461–5.
14 Ghodse AH. *Drugs and addictive behaviour. A guide to treatment,* 2nd edn. Oxford: Blackwell Science, 1995.
15 Department of Psychiatry of Addictive Behaviour. *Handbook,* 4th edn. London: St George's Hospital Medical School, 1998.
16 Lehman AF, Meyers CP, Corty E. Classification of patients with psychiatric and substance abuse syndromes. *Hosp Commun Psychiat* 1989;**40**:1019–25.
17 Department of Health. *Safety first. Five-year report of the confidential inquiry into suicide and homicide by people with mental illness.* London: DH, 2001.
18 Checinski K. Treatment strategies and interventions. In Rassool GH (ed) *Dual diagnosis. Substance misuse and psychiatric disorders.* Oxford: Blackwell Science, 2002.
19 Bien TH, Miller WR, Tonigan JS. Brief interventions for alcohol problems: a review. *Addiction* 1993;**88**:315–36.
20 Miller WR. Motivational interviewing with problem drinkers. *Behav Psychother* 1983;**11**:147–72.
21 Prochaska JO, DiClemente CC. Towards a comprehensive model of change. In WR Miller, N Heather (eds) *Treating addictive behaviours: processes of change.* New York: Plenum Press, 1986.
22 Marlatt GA, Gordon JR. *Relapse prevention.* New York: Guilford Press, 1985.
23 Department of Health. *The task force to review services for drug misusers.* London: HMSO, 1996.
24 Project MATCH Research Group. Matching alcohol treatment to client heterogeneity: Project MATCH post-treatment drinking outcomes. *J Stud Alcohol* 1997;**58**:7–29.
25 Royal College of Psychiatrists and the Royal College of Physicians. Report of a working party. *Drugs: dilemmas and choices.* London: Gaskell, 2000.
26 Health Advisory Service 2000. *The substance of young needs.* London: Health Advisory Service, 2001.
27 Ghodse AH, Tregenza GS. Drug misusers and addicts in accident and emergency

departments. In Weatherall DJ, Ledingham LGG, Warrel DA (eds) *Oxford textbook of medicine*. Oxford: Oxford University Press, 1996:4294–7.

28   Wolff K, Welch S, Strang J. Specific laboratory investigations for assessments and management of drug problems. *Adv Psychiat Treatment* 1999;5:180–91.

Useful contacts

National Drugs Helpline: Tel 0800 776600
Narcotics Anonymous: Tel 020 7730 0009
Drinkline: Tel 0800 917 8282
Alcoholics Anonymous: Tel 0845 769 7555

8 | Dementia, delirium and organic mood disorders

SUMMARY

▶ Dementia and delirium are commonly encountered in general hospitals. Both result in cognitive impairment and behavioural disturbance.

▶ Each independently affects a range of important clinical outcomes.

▶ Environmental strategies may reduce the severity of associated agitated behaviour and wandering. Improved nutritional and hydration status also reduces the incidence and severity of delirium.

▶ Medication may hamper recovery from delirium and should be used with caution. Antipsychotic drugs should be avoided because of the high risk of side effects.

▶ Many medical conditions and treatments can present with organic mood disorders.

8.1   Introduction

Dementia and delirium between them comprise a high proportion of the psychiatric illnesses presenting in general hospitals. Dementia is predominantly a disease of older people (two-thirds of general hospital beds are occupied by older people). Delirium can occur at any age, although the prevalence increases with age and with the presence of dementia. Additionally, many physical illnesses and their treatments present with symptoms which are difficult to distinguish from primary psychiatric illnesses such as depression. Consequently, general hospital staff require the core skills to diagnose dementia, delirium and depression, to initiate management and to access specialist services for more complex cases. This chapter will examine the prevalence, presentation and prognosis of dementia and delirium and will consider methods to address the associated behavioural, psychological and physical problems. Organic mood disorders will also be described.

8.2   Definition and aetiology of delirium and dementia

Dementia and delirium are syndromes reflecting the presence of an underlying pathology, rather than specific disease processes. There are similarities between them: for example, they both produce cognitive impairment and often present with behavioural manifestations. However, differentiation between the two is important, since although they are superficially similar, they have different causes and treatments.

Dementia is due to a primary or secondary disease process affecting the brain, producing a chronic, usually deteriorating, global disturbance of cognitive function.[1] Presentation depends on the stage of the illness, with a range of psychiatric, social and behavioural symptoms. The most common causes are Alzheimer's disease, vascular dementia or a combination of the two. Less common causes include dementia with Lewy body (DLB), frontotemporal dementia, Parkinson's disease, HIV infection, multiple sclerosis, Vitamin B12 deficiency and Creutzfeldt-Jakob disease. Dementia of varying severity may be encountered in general hospital patients, so it is important for staff to know how to recognise it and provide appropriate care for patients and their immediate relatives.

Delirium is an acute syndrome with a rapid onset, and is so strongly linked with an underlying physical illness that many physicians regard it as a symptom of the presence of physical illness in the same vein as chest pain or a cough. A wide variety of psychiatric symptoms and behavioural changes can occur. Delirium may be divided into hyper- and hypo-active types depending upon the overall presentation, although the fluctuating nature of delirium means that switching between the two may occur. Cardinal features are rapid onset, fluctuation, clouding of consciousness, impairment of immediate and recent memory, disorientation, perceptual disturbance, psychomotor disturbance, and alteration of the sleep–wake cycle. There is also objective evidence of underlying cause.[1]

There are numerous causes of delirium including any pathology producing infection or infarction, drug toxicity and electrolyte disturbance. Recognised independent risk factors include increased age, infection, dehydration, dementia, medications, change of location and an absence of environmental cues, particularly those which help patients orientate themselves in time and place. Many of these risk factors are common in general hospital settings.[2]

Clinical features of dementia and delirium are shown in Table 8.1. It should be noted that some dementias, particularly Lewy body dementia, may have some features of delirium (ie fluctuating cognitive and conscious state), and that chronic or subacute delirium may mimic dementia.

8.3   Prevalence

Dementia is common in general hospital populations, which is partly a reflection of the fact that older people occupy a high proportion of general hospital beds.

carers. One process used to determine whether an individual should be tagged electronically is shown in Box 8.1.

Adherence to some of these measures can be difficult; for example, the ideal situation may be a ward side-room, yet in many hospitals these are not available. The design, fixtures, fittings and decoration of many wards may increase confusion, with little in the way of orientation cues; wards must be designed and managed with dementia and delirium in mind. Effort put into training ward staff (all grades) can go a long way towards reducing the impact of illness and hospitalisation upon someone with dementia or delirium. If this is not done, staff may view these patients as being solely a psychiatric problem and may give them low priority of care.

Different approaches are required once dementia or delirium are identified. In dementia, once steps are in place to reduce incident delirium, investigations should be undertaken to detect a potentially treatable cause such as Vitamin B_{12} deficiency, hypothyroidism, or metabolic disturbance. Differentiation between Alzheimer's disease, dementia with Lewy body (DLB) and vascular dementia has become particularly important following the introduction of cholinesterase inhibitors for the treatment of Alzheimer's disease (DLB may also benefit from these drugs). The need for accurate baseline measurement of cognitive function and activities of daily living skills means that specialist services should be involved before cholinesterase inhibitors are introduced.

Box 8.1 Assessment process for electronic tagging of a confused, persistently wandering patient in a general hospital setting

If, despite:

▶ ensuring adequate hydration and nutrition

▶ optimising/minimising medication

▶ trying to ascertain why s/he is wandering (ie the purpose) and adapting to this

▶ ensuring optimal staffing levels on ward

▶ ensuring consistency of approach by staff

▶ preventing bed moves on ward

*a confused patient **persistently** wanders off the ward, then electronic tagging may be used to alert staff to the patient wandering off the ward and into potentially dangerous situations, provided:*

▶ senior ward nursing staff agree this is appropriate

▶ AND the consultant or specialist registrar also agree this is appropriate

▶ AND the patient's next of kin also agrees this is appropriate.

*The necessity for such measures **must** be constantly reviewed.*

The mainstay of management in delirium is the investigation and treatment of the underlying cause. This may be difficult in some cases, particularly where insight is impaired and behaviour is disturbed. The presence of frightening delusions and hallucinations may make gaining a patient's trust difficult. However, the treatment of the underlying cause is imperative, and in some cases detention under the Mental Health Act 1983 may be necessary to investigate and treat the physical cause of delirium. The use of a sedative drug such as lorazepam may be necessary. Antipsychotic agents should be avoided as they are potentially dangerous (especially so in hypersensitive syndromes such as DLB) and are likely to produce extrapyramidal side-effects. In delirium, antipsychotic agents are used more for their sedative effects than for their antipsychotic action, which takes up to two weeks to occur, by which time the psychotic symptoms due to delirium should have subsided as the underlying cause is treated.

A degree of tolerance to the associated behaviours such as wandering is desirable. This may be difficult to reconcile with a busy acute ward environment, yet these behaviours are commonplace and the response should not be the routine use of medication. If the wandering person is no harm to themselves or others then their behaviour should be tolerated. Attention to ward design, together with improved staff skills in non-pharmacological management, should improve the quality of care delivered. In some settings, the provision of dedicated ward environments for people with delirium and dementia can not only improve the quality of care, but also provide a useful resource for training and highlighting important skills in the management of these patients.

Dementia and delirium may be associated with other behaviours that general hospital staff find difficult to deal with. Agitation and persistent wandering may result in the use of physical restraint or involuntary sedation, where patients are not competent to consent. In this situation, restraint and treatment under common law may be necessary; however, if repeated restraint or injections are required, patients should be assessed by a psychiatrist with a view to detention under the Mental Health Act 1983. General hospitals should have a clear policy agreed with security staff for the informal restraint of patients who are at risk.

The symptoms associated with delirium are upsetting for those who experience them. Patients often have fragmented recall of events, and may suffer a post-traumatic stress reaction to the disturbing images and experiences they have undergone. Relatives and carers may also find the patient's behaviour difficult to understand. An explanation of the reasons behind these experiences, together with a warning about the likelihood of recurrence, may be beneficial to patients and relatives. Ward staff may also appreciate education and support.

9.3   Use of the medical holding order

Section 5(2) of the MHA contains a short-term holding order for 72 hours that may be used to detain an existing hospital inpatient. However, it may not be used in an A&E Department, which is regarded as an outpatient setting. Someone who is not already a hospital inpatient may only be detained under MHA sections 2, 3 or 4. Where an A&E has an associated ward, MHA section 5(2) may be applied to patients who have already been admitted to it.

Unlike patients detained under MHA section 2, 3 or 4, those held under MHA section 5(2) may not be transferred to another hospital using the authority of the MHA (in a real medical emergency it could be done under the authority of the common law) and there are no powers to treat without consent. A six-hour holding order is available under MHA section 5(4), but it may only be used by a registered mental nurse in the case of a patient already admitted for the treatment of mental disorder, so it is unlikely to be used in a general hospital.

The MHA section 5(2) power may be used by the registered medical practitioner (RMP) in charge of a patient's treatment. Once the patient is detained, the consultant has the title 'responsible medical officer' (RMO) and is the consultant in charge of the psychiatric aspects of the case. There is nothing in the MHA to confine the role of the RMO to a psychiatrist. However, given that the patient is now detained because of mental disorder, it is desirable that the medical practitioner in charge of that part of their treatment should be a psychiatrist.

In general hospitals, the initials 'RMO' are frequently applied to the resident medical officer who is usually only of senior house officer grade. It is therefore very important to be clear that, where the term 'RMO' is used in connection with the MHA, it always denotes the consultant with medical responsibility for the case.

The MHA permits the RMP to 'nominate' a deputy, who must be a registered medical practitioner (and not, therefore, a pre-registration house officer). Therefore, a consultant physician or surgeon may nominate his/her own junior as a 'nominated deputy' for the purpose of MHA section 5(2). However, it is not good practice for junior physicians or surgeons to be left to invoke the powers of section 5(2) when they and their seniors are unclear about the precise nature and scope of the powers.

The Code of Practice on the use of the MHA 1983[2] states that an RMO who is not a psychiatrist should make immediate contact with a psychiatrist when s/he has made use of his/her MHA section 5(2) power.

The MHA Commission has issued further guidance on this point for general hospitals as follows:

> It is good practice for general hospitals to have a service level agreement in place which
> allows the care and treatment for the mental disorder to be given under the direction of

a consultant psychiatrist from a psychiatric unit. Where such good practice is adhered to, the consultant psychiatrist who takes responsibility for the treatment of the mental disorder that has led to detention should be considered to be RMO for the purposes of the Act.

If a non-psychiatrist does assume responsibility as RMO, he or she should ensure that all relevant staff are aware of the implications of Part IV of the Act, which deals with consent to treatment.

Guidance can be found in Chapters 15 and 16 of the Code of Practice.[3]

9.4 Use of the place of safety order and the role of the police

MHA section 136 empowers a police constable to detain and take to a place of safety someone found in a public place who appears to be suffering from a mental disorder. This power may not be used as an emergency admission section. Its purpose is to enable someone to be assessed in safety for possible admission under the MHA. There are no statutory documents covering the MHA section 136 power, but many NHS trusts and police forces have developed their own forms to record its use.

A person should only be brought to hospital under MHA section 136 if the hospital has been designated for that purpose. In fact, in many areas it is the police station or a special area in a psychiatric unit that is a designated place of safety. A&E departments are often ill equipped for use as places of safety. They may be unsuited to receive people with severe mental disturbance and their use for that purpose may put others at great risk. In any locality, the places of safety that may be used under MHA section 136 should be agreed between NHS trusts responsible for general non-psychiatric hospitals, those that provide psychiatric services, and the police. In addition, the police should be invited to state in what circumstances they will assist in the removal of dangerous persons, and what they would do to assist hospital staff in circumstances where they have brought a dangerous person to a general hospital for medical assessment and/or care that is not available elsewhere. Police should use the A&E department for the patient if they believe this to be necessary for medical reasons (eg the patient is bleeding profusely).

9.5 Managerial arrangements for the MHA

Where an NHS trust does not normally provide inpatient psychiatric services, it may wish to make arrangements for any MHA functions to be performed on its behalf by an NHS trust that *does* provide such services. This will be particularly so for the receipt, scrutiny, and if necessary, rectification of the admission papers, and where the two NHS trusts share the same hospital site. However, even where one NHS trust delegates its functions in this way, it will still remain responsible for their performance.

Where staff of a non-psychiatric NHS trust may need to perform some MHA functions, it is important that they receive specialist training in that regard and that their performance of those functions is subject to regular, specialist review.

Non-psychiatric NHS trusts should consider issuing guidance to their clinical and security staff about the measures that may be taken, and those that are prohibited, in respect of patients who are incapable of consenting to medical treatment. Guidance will need regular review to keep abreast of changes in the law. To ensure its proper application, trusts should provide appropriate training for staff.

9.6   The common law

What is the common law?

The common law is made up of principles identified by judges as meeting the needs of particular cases. This judge-made law differs from statute law that is passed by Parliament. When the common law principles have been identified, their application to novel circumstances should follow. Common law should ideally reflect good judgement in tune with modern society; a former Master of the Rolls, Lord Donaldson, once referred to the common law as 'common sense under a wig'. Laws reflect the culture that makes them and common law can respond to new developments and shifts in the predominant cultural values of a society much more quickly than the processes that create statute law.

When does common law apply?

Common law principles may assist where there are no statutory protections or mechanisms in play. In England and Wales the Mental Health Act 1983 is the relevant codifying statute, and where its provisions apply there is little room for the common law principles. On issues where the statute law is silent, the lawfulness of any act or omission is tested by the application of the common law.

Common law principles applicable to the treatment of mentally disturbed individuals

Assumption of capacity in adults

The starting point is the recognition in common law that every adult who has reached the age of majority (18 years) has the right and capacity to decide whether or not s/he will accept medical treatment, even if a refusal may risk permanent damage to her/his physical or mental health, or even lead to premature death. The reasons for the refusal are irrelevant. Capacity is a legal concept and concerns an individual's ability to understand what is being proposed to them and the consequences of either refusing or accepting the advice given (*vide infra*). In law, pre-registration house officers are not qualified to assess a patient's capacity to accept or refuse treatment but all registered medical practitioners are.[4] Where mental disorder is present or likely, psychiatric involvement is necessary for a detailed assessment of capacity, for example in a patient who has made a suicide attempt.

The case of Ms B, a seriously physically disabled patient who wanted life-sustaining artificial ventilation turned off and who was found to have full mental capacity, has served as an example to the profession and the public of the force of this aspect of law. The judge, Dame Butler-Sloss, found that once it was established that Ms B had the necessary mental capacity to give or refuse consent to life-sustaining medical treatment, the artificial ventilation became an unlawful trespass. Moreover, if there was no disagreement about competence but the doctors were for any reason unable to carry out the patient's wishes, it was their duty to find other doctors who would do so (*The Times* Law Report, 2002).

How to assess capacity

A series of cases in the 1990s have established the principles underlying the modern general law on mental capacity. The cases described below are particularly helpful.

In *Re C*, a 68-year-old man for whom surgeons considered amputation of a gangrenous leg to be necessary to prevent imminent death, and who was already under a treatment order of the MHA for chronic schizophrenia, was judged by the court to have the mental capacity to refuse the amputation ([1994]All ER). The fact of his requiring compulsory treatment under the MHA was not evidence in itself that he was mentally incompetent to make decisions about his physical health. The judge, Justice Thorpe, adopted a three-stage test for establishing a patient's capacity to decide:

- ▶ Could the patient comprehend and retain the necessary information?
- ▶ Was he able to believe it?
- ▶ Was he able to weigh the information, balancing risks and needs, so as to arrive at a choice?

In *Re MB*, a 23-year-old woman was 40 weeks pregnant with a baby in breech position, necessitating a Caesarean section delivery (*Re MB (an adult: medical treatment)* (1997)). The woman suffered from a needle phobia and refused the Caesarean section because of anxiety about intravenous access for the anaesthesia.

After some changing of her mind she also refused anaesthesia by mask and the Caesarean section in the operating theatre. The health authority that day sought a declaration from the courts to proceed and this was granted. MB instructed her lawyers to appeal that evening, but then the following day she agreed to the procedures and a healthy baby was delivered. At the appeal against the declaration, points made by Dame Butler-Sloss with respect to capacity reiterated Lord Donaldson's earlier judgement in *Re T* that the graver the consequences of the decision, the commensurately greater the level of competence required to take the decision, and that temporary factors such as confusion, shock, fatigue, pain, or drugs may completely erode capacity, but that those concerned must be satisfied that such factors are operating to such a degree that the ability to decide is absent (*Re T (adult: refusal of medical treatment)* (1992)). Following *Re MB*, another such influence may be panic induced by fear. Again, careful scrutiny of the evidence is necessary because fear of an operation may be a rational decision for refusal to undergo it. Fear may also, however, paralyse the will and thus destroy the capacity to make a decision.

The situation for minors

People under the age of majority do not have the same rights at law as adults. It is capacity, rather than chronological age, that determines whether a child or young person can legally give valid consent to medical interventions. In England and Wales, mentally competent 16- and 17-year-olds can give consent in their own right without reference to their parents or legal guardian (Gillick competence), but their refusal can be overridden in law by parents, legal guardians or the High Court.

Best interests

After an appropriate assessment of capacity has been made, if an individual is judged to lack capacity to make the decision in question, any act or omission taken on that person's behalf must be in that person's best interests. The Law Commission[4] has recommended that, in deciding what is in a person's best interests, consideration should be given to:

▶ the past and present wishes of the individual
▶ the need to maximise as much as possible the person's participation in the decision
▶ the views of others as to the person's wishes and feelings
▶ the need to adopt the course of action least restrictive of the individual's freedom.

Best interests extend beyond purely medical considerations to incorporate broader ethical, social, moral and welfare considerations (*Re S (Adult patient's best interests)* (2000)).

Necessity

The courts have recognised the existence of a common law principle of 'necessity', and extend it to cover situations where action is required to assist another person without his or her consent. Although such a situation will usually be some form of emergency (or 'urgent necessity'), the power to intervene is not created by that urgency, but derived from the principle of necessity. In *Black* v *Forsey* (House of Lords, *The Times*, 31 May 1988), Lord Griffiths, when dealing with the common law power to restrain a dangerous mentally disordered person, said that the power was:

> confined to imposing temporary restraint on a lunatic who has run amok and is a manifest danger either to himself or to others – a state of affairs as obvious to a layman as to a doctor. Such a common law power is confined to the short period necessary before the lunatic can be handed over to the proper authority.

In common language, the judge is pointing out that it is appropriate to act to restrain patients believed to be suffering from mental disorder and who are exhibiting behaviour that suggests they are a risk to themselves or others, but where they have not yet been detained under the MHA. In practice, there is sometimes a period when patients who are about to be made subject to the MHA will have to be restrained before the formalities of the Act can be completed. It is also quite common for such patients to require some sedation prior to the completion of formalities. Such actions will be defensible if carried out as a necessity and using the minimal intervention required.

Actions performed out of necessity should not continue for an unreasonable length of time, but progress should be made either to a situation of consent or to the use of powers under the MHA. It is not possible to define precisely what is a reasonable or an unreasonable length of time, as this would vary with the particular circumstances of each case.

Duty of care

Common law imposes a duty of care on all professional staff to all persons within a hospital. By assuming the responsibility of a particular clinical staff appointment, and claiming professional expertise, an individual undertakes to provide proper care to those needing it. Staff may be negligent by omission. Actions involving the use of reasonable restraint and driven by professional responsibility in circumstances of necessity are supported by common law.

Hospital trusts themselves also have duties, for example to provide security staff who are properly trained to assist with aggressive uncooperative patients in an A&E department, and the hospital must ensure that such staff are authorised to act if necessary. Many hospitals experience problems fulfilling this duty because they fail to train security staff in this role, and such staff are often reluctant to assist in necessary restraint, as they believe that they will be exposed to the risk of litigation for assault and battery. This is a key area for improved staff training and the involvement of the trust's risk management advisers.

The Bolam test

Where clinical decisions are being made, an individual clinician's competence will be judged against what is considered reasonable and proper by a body of responsible doctors at that time, as ascertained in court from expert testimony, ie the Bolam test (*Bolam* v *Friern Hospital Management Committee* (1957)). Whilst the Bolam test remains very important, it has been modified by the House of Lords decision in the case of *Bolitho* v *City and Hackney HA* (1997), such that the decision of the doctor must be reasonable and responsible (defensible logically), or the judge may still find against.

Official guidance on consent

The Department of Health issued the *Reference guide to consent to examination or treatment* in March 2001.[5] The General Medical Council has also issued guidance on the ethical considerations with respect to seeking patients' consent,[6] and set out standards of practice expected of doctors when they consider whether to withhold or withdraw life-prolonging treatments.[7] These documents are consistent with advice given above. However, to quote the Department of Health guidance:

> *Case law on consent has evolved significantly over the last decade. Further legal developments may occur after this guidance has been issued, and health professionals must remember their duty to keep themselves informed of legal developments which may have a bearing on their practice. Legal advice should always be sought if there is any doubt about the legal validity of a proposed intervention. While much of the case law refers specifically to doctors, the same principles will apply to other health professionals involved in examining or treating patients.*[5]

9.7   The law applied to clinical cases

Having covered the principles underlying the relevant law in the jurisdiction of

England and Wales, it is helpful to consider their practical application in a number of case vignettes. All the cases have been invented for illustrative purposes. The advice given is not intended to be prescriptive, but to provide an illustration of how principles discussed in this chapter may be applied in practice. In the law, as in medicine, there is always a place for considered judgment according to the particular circumstances of each case.

CASE STUDY 1 – Acute delirium

A 54-year-old male on the high dependency unit is recovering from a cardiac arrest that required prolonged resuscitation. As he emerges from several days of coma, he becomes acutely distressed, disorientated and paranoid. He dresses himself, demands to leave and attempts to push past nursing staff. The only way to help him is to restrain and sedate him against his will, keeping him on the high dependency medical unit.

Comment – This man's refusal is not based on any real understanding of his circumstances and, in delirium, he has no grasp of his risk; it is very clearly in his best interests for him to be detained and sedated so that he can have life-saving treatments. Any reasonable lay person would not dispute this man's need for treatment and would consider hospital staff negligent if they knowingly allowed him to leave hospital.

The MHA could be applied for detention and sedation to treat the delirium (a form of mental illness), but delirium is not a condition for which the MHA is commonly used. Such patients are more often detained and treated without recourse to the MHA in view of the transient nature of the disturbance, the (so far) undisputed need for intervention and the evident lack of capacity to give meaningful consent or refusal. However, if strong measures are required to restrain him or if the situation persists over a prolonged period, it may be advisable to use the MHA. The section should be cancelled as soon as the patient has recovered mentally.

Treatments other than sedation in this case are not authorised by the MHA, but are justifiably given in a legal sense if it is judged that the patient does not have the capacity to make a meaningful refusal. The same legal decision could also apply to the use of sedation, in which case a psychiatrist need not be involved as, in law, any registered medical practitioner is considered able to judge a patient's capacity to consent.[4] This does not apply to patients detained under the MHA after the first three months of treatment; only the RMO is then judged to be able to determine a patient's capacity to consent.

CASE STUDY 2 – Patient refusing medical intervention after deliberate self-harm

A 30-year-old male is brought to A&E following an overdose of 70 paracetamol tablets taken four hours prior to arrival at hospital. There is no history available and the patient refuses to say anything about himself other than he wants to be left alone to die. He refuses to give blood for a paracetamol level and refuses any medical intervention. Can medical treatment be given without his consent?

Comment – This is a fairly common scenario. The patient presents the medical staff with the dilemma of whether they should assume he has full capacity to refuse medical treatment, in which case he might suffer the consequences of liver failure, possibly death, or whether they should act out of necessity and treat someone in whom capacity may reasonably be in doubt and where the patient could be mentally ill. The MHA does not assist with respect to treatment for the poisoning. Even where there is no formal mental illness, a patient in the state of emotional crisis surrounding attempted suicide may not be in a position to make a fully reasoned decision. Many who refuse treatment on admission are grateful for their rescue when in a calmer frame of mind the next day. In such cases physicians need to consider whether there is reasonable doubt about the patient's capacity to make a fully informed and reasoned choice in such a grave matter; if there is, they should proceed with whatever action is needed, as a matter of urgent necessity, and in his/her best interest to save his/her life. This is defensible under the common law. In the end, is it better for a clinician to have a living patient who may sue for assault and battery for saving the life they said they did not want in a highly emotional state, or to have a dead patient with grieving relatives who may sue for negligence? There are currently no exact precedents either way, but the cases of *Re T* and *Re MB* are particularly instructive (*vide supra*).

CASE STUDY 3 – Intoxicated patient refusing to cooperate with assessment following deliberate self-harm

A young adult male is brought to A&E by paramedics who found him lying in a doorway with a suicide note and an empty bottle of paracetamol. He is intoxicated with alcohol, belligerent, refuses to talk and is making moves to leave. There is no other information and staff have to make a decision as to whether or not to let him go.

Comment – This case exemplifies a common clinical problem faced by A&E staff and psychiatrists covering A&E departments. If there is sufficient concern to warrant detaining this patient for further assessment of a possible underlying mental disorder, then use of the MHA is certainly justified. The fact that the patient is intoxicated is not an obstacle to the use of the MHA, as the Act is not being used to detain or treat someone because of alcohol abuse or dependence alone (a use of the MHA excluded under Section 1(3)), but because of the concern that there may be an underlying mental disorder which is temporarily obscured by intoxication and lack of compliance.

CASE STUDY 4 – Anorexia nervosa patient *in extremis* and refusing food

A 19-year-old female with anorexia nervosa, weighing only four stones, has been admitted to the acute medical unit. She consents to a saline drip, but not to any dextrose or parenteral feeding. She is close to death from starvation.

Comment – The MHA is frequently used in relation to patients with anorexia who are close to death to authorise feeding as part of the psychiatric as well as the physical treatment of these patients. Experts in eating disorders regard re-feeding as an essential first step in the psychiatric treatment, as starvation itself produces distorted thinking. There are legal precedents to support this view, notably *Re KB*. The Mental Health Act Commission has issued guidance on this particular topic that discusses the legal issues in more detail.[8]

CASE STUDY 5 – Anorexia nervosa patient with diabetes refusing insulin

The same patient as in Case study 4 above now also has insulin-dependent diabetes; this time she agrees to feeding, but refuses insulin, since she knows she will not gain the weight without it. She would die if this plan was followed, and so the hospital staff must feed her and give her insulin if her death is to be prevented.

Comment – There is no difference between this case and the preceding situation. Insulin is as essential for healthy weight gain as food; hence its administration would also form part of the psychiatric treatment plan under Section 3 of the MHA. There is currently no legal precedent on this precise point.

CASE STUDY 6 – Patient with schizophrenia refusing surgery, but accepting other medical care

A 59-year-old male with chronic schizophrenia is a long-stay patient under Section 3. He develops a gangrenous foot and the surgeon's advice is to proceed to amputation. The patient refuses surgery on the grounds that he does not want an amputation, but he agrees to antibiotics and all other forms of treatment. The surgeon asks if the operation can be carried out as part of treatment under Section 3, as he is convinced that the patient is likely to die without the amputation.

Comment – The MHA cannot be used to authorise the treatment of the physical disorder unless it is the cause of, or as a direct result of, the mental disorder. Precedent on this [*Re C* [1994] All ER) found that a patient's gangrenous leg could not be amputated as the patient's refusal of surgery was unrelated to his chronic schizophrenia (ie he had the capacity to refuse and this refusal was not part of his psychotic thinking) and surgery would not improve his mental condition.

Acknowledgements

The working party are grateful to the Mental Health Act Commission for advice and Dr Anthony Zigmond for comments.

References

1   The Mental Health Act 1983. London: HMSO.
2   Mental Health Act Commission Guidance Note 1, 2001. *Use of the Mental Health Act 1983 in general hospitals without a psychiatric unit.* September 2001. Available on the Mental Health Act Commission website: www.mhac.trent.nhs.uk
3   Department of Health and Welsh Office (1999). *Code of practice: Mental Health Act 1983.* London: The Stationery Office.
4   British Medical Association and Law Society. *Assessment of mental capacity: guidance for doctors and* lawyers. London: BMA,1995.
5   Department of Health. *Reference guide to consent to examination or treatment.* London: DH, 2002 (www.doh.gov.uk/consent).
6   General Medical Council. *Seeking patients' consent: the ethical considerations.* London: GMC, 1999.
7   General Medical Council. *Withholding or withdrawing life-prolonging treatments: good practice in decision-making.* London: GMC, 2002.
8   Mental Health Act Commission Guidance Note 3. *Guidance on the treatment of anorexia nervosa under the Mental Health Act 1983* (issued August 1997 and updated March 1999). Available on the Mental Health Act Commission website: www.mhac.trent.nhs.uk

Further reading

Kennedy I and Grubb A. *Medical law,* 3rd edn. London: Butterworths, 2000.

Cases

Bolam v *Friern Hospital Management Committee* [1957] 2 All ER 118–128 at 122
Bolitho v *City and Hackney HA* [1997] 4 All ER 771
Black v *Forsey House of Lords, The Times,* 31 May 1988
Re B (*consent to treatment: capacity) The Times,* March 26th, 2002
Re C (*adult: refusal of medical treatment)* [1994] 1 All ER 891 (Fam Div)

Re KB [1993] 19 BMLR 144 (Fam Div)
Re MB (an adult: medical treatment) [1997] 38 BMLR 175 (CA)
Re S (adult patient's best interests) [2000] 2FLR 389 at 400
Re T (adult: refusal of medical treatment) [1992] 9 BMLR 46

Useful contact

Mental Health Act Commission
Tel: 0115 943 7100

10 | Developing a liaison service

SUMMARY

▶ Psychological problems are common in general hospital patients.

▶ Psychiatric disorders adversely affect outcomes of medical illness.

▶ In view of the effectiveness of a wide range of therapeutic interventions, liaison psychiatry services provide the best way of managing these problems.

▶ Liaison services are best managed within an acute general hospital trust, and should be based at the general hospital.

▶ Clear arrangements with commissioners are needed to ensure adequate funding.

The establishment of psychiatry and psychology services for patients in general hospitals is a relatively recent development. Services are still evolving in the light of convincing evidence of the high prevalence of psychiatric disorders in general hospital patients and of the effectiveness of a range of therapeutic interventions. Liaison psychiatry service planning and development should now be essential components of the organisational framework of care delivery in general hospitals.

10.1 The liaison psychiatry team

The psychological care for an entire general hospital is best delivered by a multi-disciplinary liaison psychiatry team based at the general hospital site. This enables close links to be developed with various medical specialties. The model operates on a consultation and liaison basis: referrals are received in response to a specific request from the referring physician but also sought proactively through the introduction of staff training and multidisciplinary meetings to improve the detection of psychiatric problems.

In addition to general services for the entire hospital, specific sessional input from psychiatry or psychology may be requested by certain medical units, thus enabling individual mental health staff to work with specific patient groups. Oncology, neurology, HIV and diabetic departments are some of the services most likely to develop links with liaison psychiatry and to fund sessions for mental health care. These links often depend on harmonious professional relationships being developed at consultant level.

Service planning should ideally be based upon epidemiological data from which the likely need can be estimated. In the general hospital setting, certain data can be used to estimate the demand. For example, the number of hospital attendances for self-harm, the percentage of general medical patients with psychiatric illness, the prevalence of alcohol problems in the general hospital setting, and rate of onset of mental illness after childbirth can all be quantified accurately. The requirements for hospitals will vary depending upon their location (inner city versus rural setting), and the size and number of specialised units. Table 10.1 shows the size of a liaison service which would be appropriate for an average general hospital with 600 beds serving a population of 250,000, based upon an estimate of likely demand.[1] A teaching hospital, serving an inner city area, with many specialised units and tertiary referral centres would require a larger service with at least two full-time consultant liaison psychiatrists. A larger rota of consultants and junior doctors would be required to provide care outside normal working hours.

Table 10.1 Estimate of size of liaison service and workload for a multidisciplinary liaison team for a district general hospital with 600 beds serving a catchment area of 250,000

Composition of liaison psychiatry service	Number
Consultant liaison psychiatrist	1
Senior house officer	1
Liaison nurses	5
Health psychologist/clinical psychologist	1–2
Secretary	1
Estimated workload	**Annual rate of patients seen**
Deliberate self-harm	500
A&E episodes	200
Ward referrals	200
Outpatient contacts	**Annual rate of patients seen**
New	100–150
Follow-up	500
Specialised liaison contacts with one or two specific units	100

10.2 Management and outcomes

What is the result of introducing more effective management of the psychological care of medical patients? The best evidence for the effectiveness of different methods of delivering high-quality psychological care of medical patients comes from the USA, where psychiatric services and interventions have been shown to reduce length of hospital stay.[2]

Where evidence is lacking, we should look for positive outcomes in a number of important areas.[3] The objectives of improving psychological care in the general hospital setting are to ensure that:

▶ earlier and better assessments are made

▶ the most appropriate advice and treatment are provided

▶ the skillmix matches the needs of patients

▶ appropriate locations for care are determined

▶ patients receive optimal care.

Based on this service philosophy, it is reasonable for a hospital considering the implementation of improvements to the psychological care of its patients to look for improved outcomes in the areas shown in Table 10.2.

10.3 Success factors

There are several important factors which lead to more successful management of psychological problems in medical inpatients. These are summarised below.

Skills and competencies of liaison psychiatry staff

Liaison psychiatry staff require a complex mix of skills, including:

▶ teamwork

▶ partnership working with other disciplines, including non-psychiatric disciplines

▶ skills of generic assessment and management of psychiatric problems

▶ skills specific to their particular professional background, such as diagnosis, psychological management and psychopharmacology

▶ clinical leadership

▶ ability to educate trainee psychiatrists and other clinical staff in the management of common problems.

Table 10.2 Outcomes potentially affected by liaison psychiatry services

Outcome	Measure(s)	Benefit
Reduced acute hospital stay	Average length of stay	Increased hospital capacity
Fewer deaths following deliberate self-harm	Mortality rates for DSH patients	Improved mental health
Reduced excess morbidity	Complication rates for defined HRGs Average length of stay	Fewer unnecessary investigations, increased inpatient capacity, improved patient satisfaction
Patient's mental health improved	Measure by survey	Fewer complaints, satisfied patients
Carer satisfaction improved	Measure by survey	Fewer complaints, satisfied carers
Staff satisfaction improved	Measure by survey, staff sickness, staff retention	Improved staff morale, improved recruitment and retention of staff
Reduced unnecessary hospital admissions	Admission rate by diagnosis Disposal rate from A&E	Improved inpatient capacity; care delivered at most appropriate location

DSH = deliberate self-harm; HRGs = high-risk groups.

Processes

It is important to consider and implement the following:

▸ The referral process should be uncomplicated with clear guidelines as to who should be referred.

▸ Protocol-guided practice: simple protocols should be developed for the detection and management of common problems by general hospital staff.

▸ There should be good channels of communication within the general hospital and with community services with regard to both psychiatric and physical health.

▸ There should be clear management structures and responsibilities. The separation of mental health and acute hospital trusts causes particular difficulties for liaison psychiatry services. This is considered further below.

10.4 Management of the service

Most psychiatric services are now managed by mental health trusts. This separation of health care provision can create difficulties for liaison psychiatry services whose therapeutic efforts are directed towards patients cared for by general hospital trusts. It is probably more appropriate for liaison services to be managed within an acute general hospital trust and to be funded from that trust's budget. Problems over resourcing have partly evolved due to management arrangements; historical models include top-sliced funding from acute trust departments, and funding from mental health trusts. It is therefore essential for the development and ongoing management of liaison psychiatry services that effective links between acute trusts and mental health trusts are established so that the development of services can be planned jointly. The establishment of a joint planning forum with shared organisational outcomes would be one means of achieving this. Both parties should clarify their priorities and identify areas of overlap and mutual interest.

10.5 Funding

Current funding of liaison psychiatry services, like so much else in the NHS, reflects historical patterns of provision at local level. The historical starting position is less important than the issues that will govern how access to funding for all NHS provision will operate in the future. Establishing how existing funding arrangements work is a good place to start, as is ensuring that there is an appreciation of the particular local commissioning arrangements. Commissioners should be made aware by acute trusts and mental health trusts of the mutual importance of liaison psychiatry services, and that provision of liaison psychiatry services should be an important part of the commissioning process. As a general guide, it would be appropriate, in considering questions of funding, to review how the service relates to the locally agreed priorities, which themselves are likely to reflect the themes identified in the NHS Plan for modernising the NHS. Establishing how a service contributes to the achievement of national or local priorities will be crucial to ensuring that funding issues are addressed.

10.6 Facilities

Wherever they are located in the general hospital, liaison psychiatry departments require adequate space for clinical work together with space for secretarial staff and support facilities to provide computerised record-keeping, thus enabling audit and clinical research to be undertaken. Mental health services for older people are beginning to appoint specialist liaison staff, similar to those developed for working age adults some 20 years ago. This is a particularly important issue, since older people occupy 60% of general hospital beds and have high levels of psychiatric comorbidity.

10.7 Research

No clinician can expect managers to develop services solely on the basis of the advice of clinicians, even when this advice comes with the seal of approval from bodies such as medical royal colleges. Evidence for clinical effectiveness is required before any new treatment is introduced or a new service is launched.

During the early days of liaison psychiatry much research was carried out to document the extent of psychiatric disorder in general hospital patients. Various groups of patients were studied in detail, particularly those consulting physicians with symptoms for which no medical explanation could be found and those with long-term, life-threatening diseases such as cancer, myocardial infarction or stroke. Little attempt was made to evaluate treatment. This omission has been rectified in recent years and there is now substantial evidence, cited in this book, for the effectiveness of various psychological and pharmacological treatments in patients with a psychiatric disorder.

10.8 Effectiveness

Doctors are also often required to demonstrate that their service is cost-effective. This is much more difficult to establish for liaison psychiatry services, since trials to demonstrate service effectiveness are expensive and difficult (though not impossible) to carry out. An effective liaison psychiatry service might reduce the cost of medical care by reducing length of hospital stay or by avoiding the use of unnecessary and expensive investigations. On the other hand, costs might be increased by virtue of increasing the numbers of patients identified and treated. We do not believe that the available evidence allows conclusions to be drawn on this topic. Until such evidence for cost-effectiveness is available, the justification for developing liaison psychiatry services should rest on their clinical effectiveness rather than on their potential to save money.

References

1   House A, Hodgson G. Estimating needs and meeting demands. In Benjamin S, House A, Jenkins P (eds) *Liaison psychiatry: defining needs and planning services.* London: Gaskell Press, Royal College of Psychiatrists, 1994:3–15.

2   Strain, JJ, Lyons, JS, Hammer JS, Fahs M *et al.* Cost offset from a psychiatric consultation-liaison intervention with elderly hip fracture patients. *Am J Psychiatry* 1991;148:1044–9.

3   Holmes J, House A. Psychiatric illness predicts poor outcome after surgery for hip fracture: a prospective cohort study. *Psychol Med* 2000;**30**:921–9.

Further reading

Department of Health. *The health of the nation: a strategy for England.* London: HMSO, 1991.

Department of Health. *National service framework for older people.* London: DH, 2001.

Department of Health. *Shifting the balance of power: securing delivery.* London: DH, 2001.